Wine

For Beginners

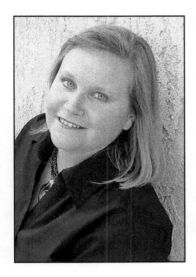

AUTHOR BIO:

Janelle Jalbert was a self-proclaimed "beer gal" until a friend's wine tasting party changed her life. Janelle's passion for wine and love of the wine lifestyle led her to become a finalist in multiple California Wine Tasting Championships just a few years after her first fateful sip. Since that time, she has visited many of the world's wine regions and has worked in various aspects of the wine industry. In addition to her other writing endeavors, Janelle continues to share her love of wine as an independent wine consultant.

Table of Contents

Introduction

"In Vino Veritas"

—Pliny the Elder, *Natural History*

"In Wine, There is Truth" is the cri de coeur of wine lovers worldwide. What exactly that truth may be if you're a little tipsy may be subject to interpretation, but one thing is true: When you drink a glass of wine, you are not only enjoying the moment you are in, but you are also connecting to generations of human beings across the millennia that have enjoyed the fruit of the vine. The wine you drink today is a distant cousin of the wine drank thousands of years ago—it is a bridge across place and time.

Wine isn't simply about drinking—it is a way to celebrate the human experience. Sure, snooty folks sometimes make it into an elitist thing with big words and odd rituals designed to create an air of superiority. But here in the real world, wine is about enjoying all that life has to offer, from marking grand moments to celebrating everyday events. It doesn't matter where you enjoy it: At a vineyard, at a fancy restaurant on a special occasion, or at your house on a Tuesday night with leftover spaghetti. Wine works with everything and for any occasion.

If you're looking for another hoity-toity wine book, this isn't it. If you want to be a wine snob or hear from one, try somewhere else. If you want to learn how to enjoy wine like you're hanging out with a chill, knowledgeable friend, you've found the right book. Welcome to *Wine for Beginners!*

The topic of wine can appear overwhelming at first, and elements of wine culture can make it seem even more out of reach, what with the special vocabulary, the rituals, and the experts who aim to make their self-anointed superiority as visible as possible. Don't lose heart: The basics are simple. You start with a bottle of wine. You open the wine. You drink the wine and decide whether you like it or not. It truly doesn't matter what others say about a particular wine. If you like it, you like it. If you don't, you don't. It is that simple.

Beyond that basic premise, wine can be as easy or as complicated as you want to make it. You can pick a random bottle and hope for the best, or just shop by whatever clever marketing trick the labelers used to get you to reach for

continued...

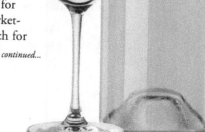

3

it. *There's nothing wrong with that.* However, the hit-and-miss approach to picking wine can get both expensive and discouraging as learn what does and doesn't work for your personal tastes. By learning a bit about how wine labels and marketing are set up, you can take some of the complications out of selecting a bottle of wine—without having to taste it first—that will delight your taste buds rather than disappoint you.

By increasing your wine knowledge, you can learn how to pick more winners than losers from the start, which will come in handy the next time you're facing bottle-packed aisles at a grocery store or a restaurant wine list that looks like a PhD dissertation written in a foreign language.

Wine does come with its own culture, which you'll learn about in this book (without the condescension.) Wine lovers have discovered and developed many beliefs and practices about how wine is to be served, what wines to serve with certain foods, and how you go about drinking wine. Why are some wines served ice cold while others at room temperature? Do you always have to have white wine with fish? What is the point of smelling the cork? Do you really have to spit out the wine at a tasting? These are some of the questions we are going to answer—and while we're at it, we'll completely debunk some myths and false claims, too.

In order to become knowledgeable about wine, you need to first understand how to select and serve a wine. Second, you need to understand how to taste a wine in a way that goes beyond whether it will get you tipsy (hint: they all will, if you drink enough.) While the second part is probably more enjoyable, the first part is necessary so that you have something in your glass that you want to drink with pleasure—rather than enduring something you hate because you've already plunked down part of your paycheck on it.

Wine for Beginners is set up to walk you through the whole process, from understanding how to pick out a bottle to actually enjoying your wine.

Here's a quick overview:

1st First, you'll get some background regarding types of wines, where they are typically found, and the regions in which specific wines are made. Regions are included here because wine drinkers often refer to a wine by a region rather than the type or varietal (you'll learn about those, too.) For example, someone may say, "This is a Bordeaux" and expect you to know what that implies. Hence, you should learn a thing or two about where certain grapes are grown.

2nd The second section covers selecting a wine, and addresses topics such as reading labels and ratings.

3rd The third topic in line is an overview of some basic wine pairings to get your own experimentations started. This section will help you understand which foods make which wines taste even better.

4th The fourth section covers the tools used to enjoy wine, including openers, glasses, and decanters. After discussing tools, the process of getting the wine into the glass is covered.

5th In the fifth section, the fun begins. That's where we start tasting wine.

Along the way, we will also cover some of the dos and don'ts in the entire process to ensure that you look like a wine rock star and not a wine dud.

If you have a hot date or another important event in the immediate future and you don't have time to read the entire book, don't sweat it: The first part is set up as a "Quick Start" guide to wine that covers the basics. Read it in combination with the Varietals section and the Wine Tasting Mechanics discussion in the Wine Tasting section. It'll give you the information you need in order to successfully "fake-it-'til-you-make-it" back to finish the book.

If you've got the time, kick back with a glass of something—anything

—and enjoy!

"*There are thousands of wines that
can take over our minds.
Don't think all ecstasies are the same!*"

—Rumi

Your Quick Start Guide

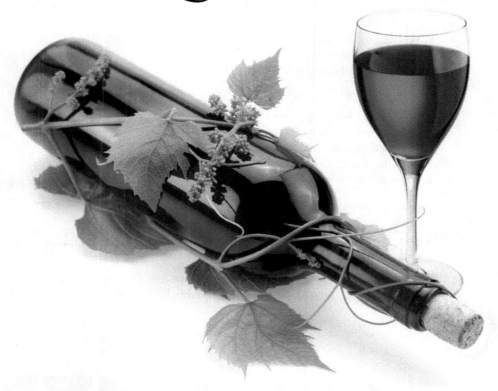

There are an estimated 10,000 varieties of wine grapes throughout the world. It would take you about 27 years to learn about all of them, if you studied one a day. That doesn't even take into account wines that are made from more than one grape. Whew!

Let's get real. There's no need to learn about all of them (unless you are going on a wine version of Jeopardy or studying to be a Master Sommelier). What's important is that you understand the major wine types and varieties that you will most likely encounter in your local store or restaurant, including where they are grown and what that means in the glass. In learning about the **types**, **styles**, and grape **varietals**, as well as where they come from, basic wine terminology also comes into play. This chapter, therefore, serves as an overview of wine types and varietals, related wine geography, and begins introducing some of the common and important wine terms.

Shop Talk...

1. **Varietals**, noun. A varietal is one of the ways in which wine is referred to—it typically denotes grapes, such as Cabernet Sauvignon and Riesling, though there is more to varietals than that (they get their own section later in the book.)

2. **Type**, noun. The descriptor used in this book for broad categories of wine using one or more varietals. Types are designated as red or white in the most general sense, but can also incorporate elements of the style in which the wine is made.

3. **Style**, noun. For the purposes of this book, a style in a sub-classification of a type of wine made with an additional factor in the winemaking process. Styles of wine include: sparkling, fortified, dessert, and so on. Also, style can refer to the way in which the wine was made in regards to how it was aged or other considerations.

What's Your Type?

Generally speaking, wines can be broken down into seven types and/or styles: **red, white, rosé, blend, sparkling, fortified, and dessert.**

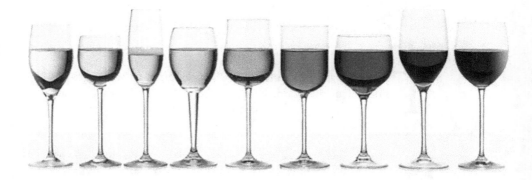

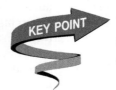 *Wines are generally referred to by either the type of wine, the style that the wine is made, or varietal of grapes used.*

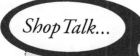

Shop Talk...

4. **Fermentation**, noun. This is the process where grape juice is made into wine. During the process, yeast and sugar turn into ethanol and carbon dioxide. The process generally takes 5 days to 2 weeks and can be completed by multiple methods.

Red versus White

The easiest distinction to make is between red and white. Red wines are created using grapes that have dark colored skins, even if the fruit inside may be a lighter color. In fact, red wine grapes can produce juice that has little or no reddish color. The level of reddish/purplish color in a wine is largely a product of the juice remaining in contact with the grape skins during the **fermentation** process. The difference between white wines and wines having a rosy to dark purple color is that the grape skins have little to no contact with the juice during the fermenting process for white and lighter colored wines.

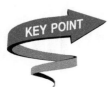

Don't be fooled. White wine can be made from both red and white grapes.

Rosés

As you may guess from the previous discussion, the pink color of rosé is the result of leaving the wine skins in the fermenting process until the pink color is achieved. An example would be White Zinfandel. There is no such thing as a White Zinfandel grape. The wine is made by pressing the Zinfandel grape, which is known to be a darker color, and letting the pressed and settled juice mix with the skins to achieve the color and taste of White Zinfandel.

The benefits for this "halfway" process are not simply about producing a pink wine. The darker skins also change the taste of the wine itself. Rosé wines have a taste that is richer than a white version but with a lower level of **tannins** than a fully red wine. Rosés are a product of the fermentation process, not blending.

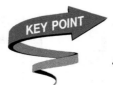

Rosés are not blends of white and red wine. The color comes from limited contact with grape skins during fermentation.

Blends

Don't get confused now that you've learned rosé is not a blend—blended wines do, in fact, exist. A blended wine will most likely be between wines of the same type: all reds or all whites. They are the product of combining the juice of two or more varietals. The combinations create wines with different flavors, aromas, textures, and alcohol content. The goal in making a blend is to a wine that is flavorful and unique—it is not, as the myth goes, to "water the wine down."

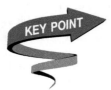

The concepts of a blended versus varietal wine can be deceiving. A bottle of Cabernet Sauvignon does <u>not</u> have to be 100% Cabernet Sauvignon.

Wine laws variety from place to place, and the definition of a blended wine changes as well. In the United States, there are many different rules. In California, where the majority of American wines are made, a wine is considered a "blend" if it has less than 75% of any single varietal in it. If it has at least 75% of a particular varietal, it can be labeled as a single varietal. So in California, you might buy a bottle of Cabernet Sauvignon that is 82% cabernet and 18% other grapes, for instance. However, things get confusing fast when you take into account that these rules vary from state to state. Just a little north in Oregon, a bottle of Pinot Noir must be 90% pinot to be labeled as such.

The truth is that a bottle of wine is rarely 100% of a single varietal, but exactly how much depends on the region in which it was grown.

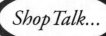

Shop Talk...

5. **Tannins**, noun. The bitterness in a wine as the result of the wine seeds, skins, and stems coming into contact with the wine during fermentation. Tannins are what make wine taste dry and biting. Outside of wine, a taste example of tannins is bite that comes with unsweetened black tea.

Sparkling

Let's take a minute here and clear something up: Bubbly is not bubbly. Some folks mistakenly refer to all sparkling wines as Champagne, regardless of where the wine was made. That is a huge no-no.

For a long time, the only wine that was labeled "Champagne" was from grapes grown in the French region of—wait for it—Champagne. An American judge recently ruled that any sparkling wine could be marketed as "Champagne" in the United States, which royally upset the French—and which most wine lovers also turned their noses up at. My advice to you is to reserve your use of the term "Champagne" only for sparkling wines made in the French Champagne region. If it came from anywhere else, call it "sparkling wine" instead.

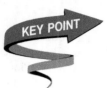 *The term "Champagne" only refers to sparkling wines produced in the French region of Champagne.*

Sparkling wines also have an added level of classification based on the level of sugar present in each liter of wine. This is a characteristic that is unique to sparkling wines.

Here's a quick list of those terms:

- ▶ **Brut Zero** = 0 grams
- ▶ **Brut Nature** = 0-3 grams
- ▶ **Extra Brut** = 0-12 grams
  (Greatest degree of variation in sweetness of all sparkling wines)
- ▶ **Extra Dry** = 12-17 grams
- ▶ **Dry** = 17-32 grams
- ▶ **Demi-Sec** = 32-50 grams
- ▶ **Doux** = 50+ grams

The most important terms to know are "dry" (we'll get into that later, as it applies to many different wines) and specifically with sparkling wines, Extra Brut. This is the classification with the biggest range in sweetness. Extra Brut can include wines with anywhere from a few grams of sugar all the way up to 17 grams per liter. Extra Brut is in the low to midlevel of sweetness when it comes to sparkling wines.Sparkling wines such as Champagne, Prosecco, Asti Spumante, and Cava are wines that have undergone a secondary fermentation process to develop bubbles in the wine. The extra fermentation process allows for yeast to consume the sugars, and the bubbles result from the "burping off" of carbon dioxide in the process.

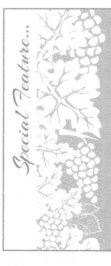

Casks

Casks range from large vats to barrels, in which wine fermentation and aging occurs. They are typically made of wood or steel. The use of either material impacts the nature of the wine produced. Steel tends to produce a wine that has more floral and fruit (like apple) notes, while wood creates deeper notes like vanilla, caramel, smoke, and spice. Wood is often used with red wines to also help mellow out some of the tannins present.

Champagne undergoes the first round of fermentation in a wooden cask. The secondary fermentation is done in the bottles themselves. Champagne can only be made from a combination of three grapes: Chardonnay, Pinot Meunier, and Pinot Noir. (You'll learn more about Chardonnay and Pinot Noir later in this part of the book.)

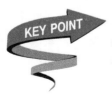

Casks range from large vats to barrels, in which wine fermentation and aging occurs. They are typically made of wood or steel.

Traditions regarding the creation of sparkling wines can differ outside of France. Prosecco and Asti Spumante are tied to Italian winemaking, while Cavas are from Spain. All have a degree of bubbliness to them. Sparkling wines from these other regions can be made in either wood or steel casks, unlike French Champagne, which must be fermented in wood. The Spanish Cava is made from the Macabeu grape. Italian sparkling wines are regulated by the government: Asti Spumante (or simply Asti) must be made of only the Muscato Bianco grape, whereas Prosecco is from the Glera grape. Traditionally, Prosecco is served only in spring, while Asti, Champagne and other sparkling wines are served year-round.

Realistically, it's not particularly important to know the different varietals used in sparkling wine. For practical purposes, the critical element involves the size and nature of the bubbles. Smaller and slower moving bubbles indicate a higher quality wine because smaller bubbles allow for more aromatics to get trapped inside the wine. Smaller bubbles also indicate a more natural fermentation process during production because larger bubbles are usually the result of extra carbon dioxide being pumped into the wine (which is usually how soda is carbonated.)

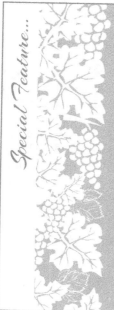

Special Feature...

What's the Riddle in Sparkling Wine?

Riddling is not about a play on words. Riddling (or Le Remuage) in winemaking is the process of turning the bottles of sparkling wine. Higher quality sparkling wines are aged in the bottle after the first fermentation. This means additional time from vine to the table (and usually means a higher price tag too). It also requires the services of a "riddler" who turns the bottles 1/8th of a turn each day during the secondary fermentation process.

Talk about carpal tunnel syndrome—a typical riddler turns 20,000 to 30,000 bottles a day!

Port/Fortified Wines

Fortified wines are a special class of still (not sparkling) wines that are "fortified" with a spirit. Hence, the process of fortification is used to enhance the wine's body, flavor, and ageability. The most common fortification is brandy. The process was originally created as a way of increasing storage options in the 17th and 18th centuries as ocean exploration and conflict required that wine be made to last for long voyages or campaigns.

Shop Talk...

6. **Fortification**, noun. The process of adding a distilled spirit to a wine to "fortify" it. Fortified wines include: Ports, Sherries, Madeira, Masala, and some Vermouths.

For our purposes, we will focus on Ports (they're capitalized because they're short for Porto, a town in Portugal.) Port wines are the most widely known style of fortified wine. The most common Ports are reds, but there is

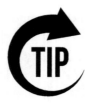

Vintage ports do not happen every year.
Traditionally, a vintage may only
be declared in a few different years
of any one decade.

a growing market for white Ports, too. Ports are often designated by the way they are aged. Wood-aged ports are designed to be consumed at a younger age while bottle-aged ports are intended to take a decade or more to fully develop and mature. Ruby Ports are the youngest, with an average of 3 years of aging, and have a notable red color. The Tawny Port is a deeper red than the Ruby and has a nuttier flavor. Tawnies are most often designated by age with labels of 10, 20, or 30 years. The most elite are Vintage Ports, which are made from the best of the best grapes in a given year. Vintage Ports are designed to age 20 years or more before drinking.

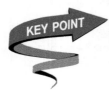

Fortified wines contain the addition of distilled spirits, most often brandy.

Dessert Wines

Dessert wines are a broadly defined type of wine that is typically sweeter but can include wines from other categories such as late harvests of different varietals, Ports, and Moscato d'Asti. The "purest" dessert wines include Ice Wines, Raisin Wines (such as Vin Santo in Italy), and Noble Rot Wines. These are super sweet, often syrupy, versions of wine.

Dessert wines have a special marketing practice related to their content and pricing. These wines are often sold in smaller 375ml bottles compared to the standard 750ml bottle. There are two reasons for this. One, the cost of producing such wines is much higher because of time on the vine for ripening and other factors, so the smaller bottle is more economical. Two, dessert wines are so much sweeter that the standard glass pour is approximately 2 oz. rather than 6 oz.

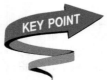

Dessert wines are usually sold in smaller bottles due to cost and high levels of sweetness.

Noble Rot, Not All Bad for Wines

Noble Rot may sound like a situation that should send you to the drugstore for medicine, but in wine it is considered positive—it helps create some of the sweetest wines on the market. Botrytis Cinerea (the scientific name for Noble Rot) is a mold that grows on grapes in vineyards under certain conditions. The mold dehydrates the grape while on the vine and shrivels the fruit up like raisins, concentrating sugars (and thus flavors) to much higher levels. Wines using Noble Rot include Sauternes from France and some versions of German Rieslings.

While wines produced with Noble Rot use grapes that appear to have become raisins on the vine, true raisin wine utilizes heat shrivel to grapes, concentrating their flavors and sugars. The most recognizable type of raisin wine is Italy's Vin Santo. Despite interesting stories about how this "Holy Wine" got its name, the process of making it remains as simple as it was in the 1300s when it first went into production. Winemakers take the best bunches of grapes and dry them on racks before putting the juice in small casks for a long period of aging. There are no vintages for such wines, but they are ready for immediate drinking, as well as able to hold up for almost indefinite aging.

Ice wines are the cold weather counterparts to raisin wines and Vin Santo. In order to make Ice Wine, grapes are allowed to remain on the vine late into the season until they freeze. The process works in the same manner as Noble Rot and drying. The grapes become dehydrated, so the flavors and sugars are concentrated. For obvious reasons, Ice Wines are typical in areas of colder weather. Germany (Ice Wine is called Eiswein there—it's pronounced the same) and Canada are the largest producers. New York also has a growing reputation for its Ice Wines. In France, some wine producers replicate freezing within their cellars to achieve similar results.

Author's Aside

With so much already covered—and we've only discussed the types of wines—I can sympathize if your mind is already spinning. There's a lot to process.

I was a certified "Beer Only Gal" when I was invited to my first wine tasting party. The only wine I had before that invitation was a very rare glass at a wedding. I was assigned to bring a bottle of Gewürztraminer. My immediate response was "A Ga-What?" The host swore it was an easy grocery store find for someone as clueless as I was. Yeah, right. I went to three stores on my first venture into the wine aisles, never asked for help until I went to a specialty wine store, and ended up with a $20 bottle when a $6 one would have been just fine. Live and learn.

It does get easier. Trust me. Hang in there. We're about to learn about the varietals, so you'll be better off than I was when I showed up to my first wine experience.

Varietals: Just the Basics

We started the section with the staggering fact that there are more than 10,000 varieties of wine grapes throughout the world. There is really no need to be familiar with them all. The most you need to master is four whites and five reds to get started. The rest is gravy. You can always do your own research, both through books and experience, to learn about the others, but nine is the ticket in the door.

Author's Aside

Covering the core varietals is as much about the experience as it is about the book learning of what to expect. For the quickest, easiest, and probably most fun way to understand the following section which talks about how each wine tastes and smells, I would suggest having a taste of each wine (or at least a couple of them) to put the words and tastes together at the same time. If you're near a wine bar, restaurant, or store that has tastings, take this book with you and don't be shy about asking questions of those who work there or who are more experienced wine drinkers. There's one thing that is nearly a guarantee: Wine drinkers love to talk about wine.

At first, the core varietals may look and sound like foreign language (most of them are,) but with a little practice they will roll off your tongue easily. On the white end of the wine spectrum, the core varietals are Pinot Gris, Chardonnay, Riesling, and Gewürztraminer. The red wines to be familiar with are Pinot Noir, Merlot, Zinfandel, Cabernet Sauvignon, and Syrah.

Here's a quick guide to pronouncing the core varietals:

White Wines

Pinot Gris (pronounced "Pee-no Gree") or
Pinot Grigio (pronounced "Pee-no Gree-gee-oh")

Chardonnay (pronounced "shar-dawn-AY")

Gewürztraminer
(pronounced "guh-VURTS-trah-mee-ner")
The W is pronounced as a V in line with the Germanic roots.

Riesling (pronounced "REEZ-ling")

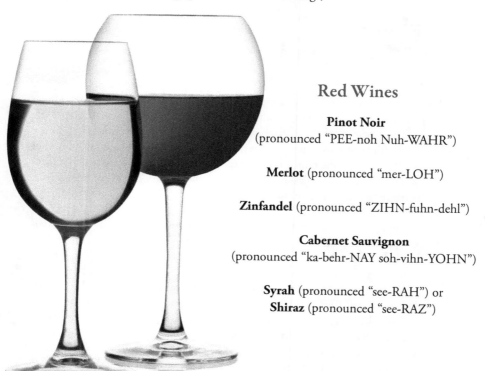

Red Wines

Pinot Noir
(pronounced "PEE-noh Nuh-WAHR")

Merlot (pronounced "mer-LOH")

Zinfandel (pronounced "ZIHN-fuhn-dehl")

Cabernet Sauvignon
(pronounced "ka-behr-NAY soh-vihn-YOHN")

Syrah (pronounced "see-RAH") or
Shiraz (pronounced "see-RAZ")

Core White Wines

Pinot Gris/Pinot Grigio

Pinot Gris and Pinot Grigio are white wines that come from the same grape, which is a grayish-red fruit. When it comes to labeling wines by varietal, they are considered to be the same. However, when the wine's style is considered, the two wines have distinct characteristics due to where the grapes are grown and the winemaking process, which accounts for the different names. It is part of the Pinot family of grapes, which includes both white and red wines. The term "pinot" is French for "pine cone," the shape that characterizes the grape clusters in the family of varietals. Pinot Gris terminology reflects the wine's French roots while Pinot Grigio reflects the touch of Italian influence on wine produced from the varietal.

More ardent wine drinkers often argue about the nature of the Pinot Gris/Pinot Grigio debate. It is more a question of labeling expectations. For those who want a light and refreshing version of this grape, Pinot Grigio is the answer. If a drinker wants a fuller and lingering taste in the mouth from the wine, then Pinot Gris is the way to go.

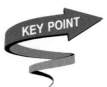

Pinot Gris and Pinot Grigio are from the same grape. Gris is a fuller wine from France, and Grigio is a lighter wine from Italy.

Regardless of whether it's gris or grigio, white wine made from Pinot grapes is known for citrusy and fruity flavors, depending on the level of ripeness of the grapes at harvest. Younger grapes will give hints of lime, green apple, and sometimes some pear note. On the Pinot Grigio end of the spectrum, the wine tends to be lighter in color, from nearly white to a pale yellow. More mature grapes and wines on the Pinot Gris side of things will provide flavors of lemon, honeysuckle, and nectarine.

Pinot Gris and Pinot Grigio are typically fermented in steel casks which emphasize the citrus and green apple components. There is a refreshing level of acidity that is balanced with a natural minerality, which is viewed as a basic characteristic of the varietal. This fact makes Pinot Gris and the even lighter Pinot Grigio popular wines for warm-weather drinking. The lightness and dryness of the Pinot Gris wine is balanced with a weightier feel on the tongue and in the mouth which provides a satisfying drinking experience while maintaining lightness. Unlike Riesling, both of these lighter white wines can be labelled as dry wines because of a lower level of sweetness. These wines are suited for drinking alone as well as with lighter food dishes because of the softer levels of tannins present.

Shop Talk...

7. **Dry**, adj. This means that there is no residual sugar in the wine leftover after fermentation. People often confuse the terms "dry" and "sweet" in wine with elements of acid or tannins. We will discuss this point further in the "Wine Tasting" section.

Pinot Gris from the French region of Alsace is among the most complex wines produced with this grape and has a typical taste profile that includes lemon and honey combined with notes of spices like cinnamon, ginger, and clove. The finish, or aftertaste and mouth feel, for these types of Pinot Gris is long lasting and maintains a tingly feeling on the tongue and in the mouth. American Pinot Gris and Pinot Grigio is more of a blend of the two other versions, with less acid and more over-the-top fruit flavors. For this reason, Pinot Gris and Pinot Grigio are often viewed in America as an easy, "entry type," variety for those starting to drink wine.

Shop Talk...

8. **Finish**, noun. The aftertaste that lingers in the mouth after the wine has been swallowed. A long finish of 30 seconds or more is considered a positive characteristic of wine.

Chardonnay

Now, we come to the "big one" of white wines. The Chardonnay grape is the most planted white wine grape in the world. It is also the most popular wine, red or white, in the United States. It is a versatile grape with a wide range of aroma and flavor profiles. The wine produced from Chardonnay grapes can reflect both the growing conditions and the production process to create a unique drinking experience that can make bottles taste different from one winery to the next, even in the same region. It is one reason the varietal has come to be known as the "winemaker's wine."

Despite the diversity of Chardonnay, the wine from this varietal falls into four general categories. The first three categories are fruit based while the fourth is based on oak aging. The most common taste and scent categories involve apple and pear notes. Chardonnays do not have the more common citrusy characteristics of other white wines, but when citrus is present it is in the form of lemon, orange, and grapefruit. The final fruit category for Chardonnay is tropical, which includes melon, pineapple, and banana. These Chardonnays tend to be made in steel vats as opposed to wooden barrels.

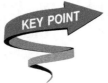

Chardonnay wines are often characterized by the use of steel or oak during fermentation which can make the wine taste fruitier or more buttery.

Flavor is also imparted to Chardonnay wines based on the fermentation and aging process. Chardonnay is regularly described by the way in which it was processed: oak casks or steel vats. Steel Chardonnays lean towards the green apple and citrus notes. Oak Chardonnays have an added level of flavor and scent with notes of oak (obviously), butter, smoke, spice, and vanilla. Also, if the winemaker chooses to leave the wine in contact with the skins, seeds, and such for a longer period following fermentation, the wine will develop a deeper aroma and flavor profile that can include elements of a doughy bread smell and taste. The presence of these elements does not make the Chardonnay "better" or "worse." It is a matter of personal preference when deciding between a buttery/oaky Chardonnay, a green apple/citrusy wine, or something in between.

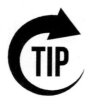

While your choice of Chardonnay flavor profile is a matter of preference, there are times when a wine with specific characteristics will be a better choice. This is especially important when pairing food with Chardonnay. If you want the skinny right now, jump ahead to the "Wine Pairing" section.

Gewürztraminer

Now we reach the infamous "Ga-What?" grape that I mentioned earlier. It is the easiest wine to identify from a taste perspective and the most challenging to spell. Gewürztraminer translates into "Spicy Grape," and lives up to its reputation. This is a varietal that produces a love/hate relationship for wine drinkers. Those who love it enjoy the spice and uniqueness. Those who hate it dislike the low acid and powerful fruit characteristics. Whatever you feel about it, Gewürztraminer is the easiest wine to learn to identify.

Gewürztraminer grapes are pink-skinned and grow in cooler regions. The Alsace region of France is the one most associated with the varietal, but the wine is also produced in Germany, Italy, New Zealand, Washington, Oregon, and cooler areas of California.

The most notable scents associated with Gewürztraminer are floral (especially rose petal), peach, spice, lychee and citrus. When it comes to taste, Gewürztraminer includes a combination of fruits such as apricot, peach, and mango (otherwise known as "stone fruits") with the spice of cinnamon and ginger. In some cases, the floral notes can be intense enough to be tasted as well as smelled.

Author's Aside

On a trip to the Northern California coast, I took a lengthy cruise off of Highway 1 on a logging road to the incredible Annapolis winery. As I tasted their Gewürztraminer, the rose hitting my nose and palate lit me up. It was balanced with apricot and spice and was downright amazing. They had mistakenly poured the upcoming vintage instead of the current one, but the mistake worked for both sides: Though it wasn't for sale yet, I walked out with a case at the previous year's prices, and they realized they had a more special wine to market then they first thought. Trust me, those types of wine finds are always the most fun and memorable.

Riesling

This fruity and sometimes sweet wine is something of the opposite of Chardonnay on the white wine color spectrum, but it can be as diverse in range of flavors. It is lighter and not associated with the influence of oak, but don't let that fool you. In terms of complexity and versatility, Riesling rivals Chardonnay. Rieslings are often misunderstood for being only sweet in nature, but the wines from Alsace (France), Germany, and some areas of the United States can be dry and very complex.

Rieslings are known for intense fruit flavors. Apricot, pineapple, citrus, honey, and floral notes are the most recognizable characteristics of this varietal. The acidity of Riesling gives it a crispness that balances out the sweetness. This balance allows Rieslings to be sweet without being syrupy, unless the wine is designed to have a thick sweetness typical of late harvests and dessert wines. Because of the characteristic balanced sweetness in Rieslings, this wine is a good "starter wine" for those with little wine experience or who favor White Zinfandel but want to broaden their knowledge.

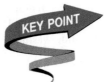

Riesling is a common varietal for late harvest wines. This can lead to the misconception that all Rieslings are super sweet, which is not true.

Riesling wines from Germany and Washington State tend to be dry and crisp when not done in a dessert style. While most Washington State Rieslings are meant to be enjoyed young, those from Germany can be aged for 5 to 10 years to develop fully. The German classifications for the wine can be a bit daunting for those new to Riesling and not familiar with German. The classes are based on the level of sweetness in the wine. The driest German Riesling is Kabinett followed by Spätlese, which is slightly sweeter. The midrange on sweetness is the Auslese class with Beerenauslese a touch sweeter. The Trockenbeerenauslese is the most intense and sweetest, and is often considered a dessert wine.

Is it critical to know how to pronounce each of these terms? Heck no—you don't even need to remember them. In reality, unless you are targeting a dry versus sweet German Riesling for a specific purpose, the terminology is just a bonus. If you find yourself at a wine store hunting down German Rieslings, these are good to know, but knowledgeable staff should be able to point you in the right direction and no one you're clinking glasses with is going to look down on you for forgetting "Trockenbeerenauslese" (because they probably will, too.)

Author's Aside

The only time I was at a loss for the terminology was during a trip to Germany when I was looking for a sweet Riesling to bring home to mom. Then, I was lost and had to make the sacrifice of tasting several to figure it all out. (Yeah, the sacrifices we make for family.)

If you are looking to try Riesling and don't want the headaches of the German terminology, you can stick with wines made in the United States. The labels will be straightforward in telling you if it is dry or sweet or even a late harvest.

While there are thousands of white wine varieties, knowing about Pinot Gris/Pinot Grigio, Chardonnay, Gewürztraminer, and Riesling provides you with a solid foundation about white wines. You can rest easy knowing these four varieties, or you can view it as the platform from which you can dive into further exploring white wines.

Core Red Wines

Let's pivot to the red side of the spectrum. The four "need to know" red wines are Pinot Noir, Merlot, Cabernet Sauvignon, and Syrah. These are arranged in order of intensity, so if you are new to red wines you may want to start with Pinot Noir and work your way through the list. However, a good Merlot is a fine starting point for a more universal red wine pairing with dishes. We will discuss food pairings in a later section. First, let's understand the wines themselves.

Pinot Noir

Pinot Noir is a bit of a chameleon and diva of a wine. It is at the lightest and most subtle end of the red wine spectrum for appearance and taste. Given that fact, Pinot Noir can be enjoyed with some foods that are typically associated with white wines instead of reds. The wine can be a challenge to both grow and appreciate. The vines themselves are relatively weak and prone to disease and mutations. The climate Pinot Noir thrives in is strictly defined, with vines needing warm days and cool nights to properly develop. Done right, Pinot Noir can have great subtlety in bouquet and flavor or can be quite pronounced in smell and taste. Recognizing the range in the final Pinot Noir product is often seen as a challenge to those who would present themselves as wine snobs. The perception of elitism combined with the production considerations can make some bottles of Pinot Noir more expensive in comparison to other red varietals.

The flavor of a Pinot often is in line with the color of the wine. Lighter Pinot Noirs highlight strawberry and red cherries in their bouquet and flavor. Darker, deeper Pinot Noirs have hints of black cherry and leather. Pinot Noir, especially the dark versions, are also known for hints of terroir and sous-bois, which give the wine an earthy flavor.

Shop Talk...

9. **Terroir**, noun or adjective. Pronounced tare-WAHR, the term comes from the French word for land, terre. The concept of terroir involves a sense of the place where the specific vine grows within a wine. "Place" is reflected in the glass through the bouquet and flavor of the wine. Elements of minerals, soils, nearby vegetation, and climate can be tasted as a wine's terroir. Examples include: hints of lavender in wines from the South of France, the bolder and fruiter California Pinot Noir compared to its earthy cousin from the colder Burgundy region, and hints of limestone and other minerals present from a particular wine region.

Pinot Noir is a key element in the production of most sparkling wines, be it white or the pink version, which is known as Blanc de Noirs ("white from black," referencing a white wine made from black grapes.) We'll cover more details about Pinot Noir's role in sparkling wines a little later in the book.

Shop Talk...

10. **Sous-Bois**, noun and adjective. Pronounced soo-BWAH, this is a term used most often with French Pinot Noir, especially from Burgundy. It refers to a vegetative note in the wine (the word means "undergrowth" in French.) No, we aren't talking about weeds and grass here (though there are varietals known for a grassy note). This is more of a forest-floor aroma and taste; think notes of mushrooms or truffles in the glass or on the tongue, and a damp soil smell or taste. It is not a flaw in wines.

Merlot

In years past, commercialization and lower quality standards led to Merlot's reputation as an inferior wine. The fact is that Merlot is the most planted grape variety in France. It is enjoyed as both a top-rated, stand-alone varietal as well as a key element to red wine blends that require more balance. The tannin levels are usually lower than those found in Cabernet Sauvignon, making it friendly to newer wine palates. Lighter tannins make Merlot a wine that can be enjoyed on its own, as well as one that pairs easily with food. Merlot hits the midrange of the spectrum for both color and body among red wines, making it more accessible than wines at either extreme. The fruit in Merlot is emphasized rather than the tannins, so it lacks the structure or ageability of Cabernet and other reds. Thus, Merlot is enjoyed sooner rather than later when consumed in a single varietal bottle. It is also one of the major reasons that wine drinkers view Merlot as inferior to other red varietals.

Merlot, more than most varietals, illustrates the impact of climate on the finished product. Cool weather Merlots produced in Bordeaux, other regions in France, and around Italy tend to have a higher tannin level with more terroir influences and flavors like plum, licorice, berry, currant, anise, tobacco, and coffee. Even tar and charcoal tastes can be present! These wines have longer finishes, meaning they last longer in your mouth between sips and are more full-bodied. Merlots from warmer areas like California, Argentina, and Australia tend to be sweeter with more mellow tannin structures to provide a rounded, silky, and generous feel in the mouth. These Merlots have less acid than their cooler cousins. The flavors that stand out for a warm-weather Merlot include cherry, raspberry, cocoa, floral, spice, and mocha. The warmer weather wines are easily enjoyed as a stand-alone drink, while the cooler Merlot versions are primed to be combined with food for the best drinking experience.

Zinfandel

If there was such a thing as an "American" wine, Zinfandel would be it. Though not limited to the United States, Zinfandel is associated most with the United States. Ten percent of California vineyards, especially along the Central Coast, are under Zinfandel vine. California has approximately three times more "Zin" (the abbreviated reference for Zinfandel) than its nearest competitor. In other regions—such as Puglia, Italy and Croatia—Zinfandel is also known as Primitivo. Zinfandel is lighter in color than Merlot and Cabernet Sauvignon but can pack a wallop when it comes to the level of alcohol present. The alcohol content by volume (ABV) on Zinfandels can be in the 14%-17% range compared to other wines in the 10%-12% range. Zinfandel's moderate tannin levels and high acidity, combined with higher alcohol levels, can produce an oily texture in the mouth. These big "in-your-face" characteristics help contribute to the wine world's association between American interests and Zinfandel.

In addition to the elements of alcohol and tannin, a glass of Zinfandel is regularly characterized by hints of cherry, blackberry, currant, raisin, and plum on the nose. Medium- and full-bodied Zinfandels have elements of oak, vanilla, chocolate, coffee, tobacco, smoke, and black or white pepper. In the mouth, the flavors and the bouquet can produce an additional experience of cedar, spice, and earthy notes.

While Zinfandel is a red wine with a big reputation, White Zinfandel is one of the most recognized types for those new to wine. To some wine snobs, White Zinfandel doesn't warrant mentioning, but the pale pink version of Zinfandel makes up more than 80% of all Zinfandel production. White Zinfandel is made with the same grapes as "traditional" Zinfandel. The only difference between the red and white versions of Zinfandel is the amount of time the grapes' juices remain in contact with the grapes' skins during the fermentation process. A shorter contact time makes the resulting wine is more pale, and lower in tannin levels. White Zinfandel lacks the complexities of the red version because of this practice. However, lower alcohol levels (averaging approximately 10% ABV) and increased sweetness make White Zinfandel a popular entry-level wine.

Author's Aside

Technically, White Zinfandel would be considered a blush wine or a rosé, but those new to wine need to understand that White Zinfandel is not a separate grape. Yes, I have been at wineries where visitors saw rows of labeled vines and asked, "Where's the White Zinfandel?" Often the question came while they were standing next to a row of Zinfandel vines. At least now, you won't be the one making such a faux pas, so go ahead and let the snobs cringe at the White Zinfandel in your glass. If you enjoy it, that's all that matters.

Cabernet Sauvignon

Cabernet Sauvignon will often be referred to as "Cab," despite several Cabernet varietals, or "Cab Sav," so don't let the shorthand fool you into missing this important wine. Cabernet Sauvignon is one of the most planted vines and most popular wines. Ironically, this powerhouse varietal is actually an unlikely combination of other varietals. The varietal was tested at UC Davis in 1996. Cab DNA revealed it was actually a cross between the Cabernet Franc (a red varietal) and Sauvignon Blanc (a white varietal) that is believed to have naturally combined sometime in the 17th century. Cabernet Sauvignon is lighter than a Syrah though the tannins and acidity in a Cab can range from a medium to high level.

Cabernet Sauvignon is a full-bodied wine that has several elements of aroma and flavor that make it different from other red varietals. It is aged in a combination of different types of oak barrels, so it is no surprise that oak is common in the bouquet and taste. Each type of oak used, French or American, gives the wine a distinct flavor. The smell and taste of a Cabernet Sauvignon share similarities with a Zinfandel with notes of black cherry, blackberry, black pepper, tobacco, vanilla, and cedar. Differences between Zinfandel and Cabernet Sauvignon include the previously mentioned oak, as well as licorice, and even bell pepper. Geographical influences, related to where the grapes are grown, can also come through in the wine. French Cabernets can have hints of mint, graphite, and gravel. Cabernets from Australia can include eucalyptus and menthol notes. Cabernet Sauvignon grown in hotter environments can also taste "jammy" because of the grapes being over-ripened, while cooler growing conditions can give the wine hints of black olives and green pepper.

Special Feature...

What Do Ladybugs and Bell Peppers Have in Common?

They both impart unique characteristics, read as flaws, to Cabernet Sauvignon.

All Cabernet Sauvignon grapes have pyrazines, which are molecules containing nitrogen with hydrogen and carbon, but under-ripened grapes have the highest levels. Sunlight destroys pyrazines as grapes mature. Since cooler climates do not benefit from as much sun exposure, the pyrazines can survive all the way into the bottle. The result? The wine ends up smelling and tasting like green pepper. Canadian winemakers dumped more than a quarter of a million gallons of wine down the drain in 2001 because of the overpowering smell of bell pepper, asparagus, peanuts, and such when grapes were harvested. It wasn't simply because of the pyrazines present in Cabernet Sauvignon, it was because of a thing called "Ladybug Taint." In this case, the polka-dotted beetles are no friend to a wine drinker. Ladybugs have a version of a pyrazine in their bodies, and researchers realized that if the friendly-looking critters were still present when the harvested grapes went to crush, they "poisoned" the whole batch in remarkable ways. Gary Pickering, a wine professor at Brock University, says that humans are extra sensitive to ladybug pyrazines - a single drop of it can ruin an Olympic-size pool of wine for us. That amount is equal to an entire vine being sabotaged by single ladybug that got caught in the harvest. Ick, I'll take my wine ladybug free, please!

A bottle of 100% Cabernet Sauvignon is a rarity because it is commonly used to blend with other varietals. Super Tuscans in Italy are a blend using primarily Cabernet Sauvignon and Sangiovese, and Bordeaux wines are primarily Cabernet Sauvignon that are softened with other varietals such a Merlot.

Author's Aside

Life is a Cabernet, at least for a day. Need an excuse to pop the cork on a bottle of Cab? Thanks to a 2010 marketing stunt that went viral, the last Thursday in August is now Cabernet Day. Cabernet-themed events are held worldwide on that day. The celebration often continues into the following weekend as well. If you are interested, the event is promoted under #CabernetDay in social media. Cheers!

Syrah

Syrah, or Shiraz as it is named in Australia, is the darkest of the reds we discuss here, and has a reputation for being both accessible and quite elite. If Zinfandels are "big and bold," Syrah kicks it up a notch to "big, bold and bad." That's "bad" in a good way. Syrah is a "big, bad, barbecue wine" on one end of the spectrum and a sophisticated foundation for the celebrated Rhône wines of Southern France at the other end. Tannin and acidity levels can range from medium to high with the nose and taste influenced by oak aging.

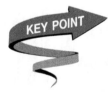 *Syrah is referred to as Shiraz in Australian wines.*

It is also important to note that Syrah and Petite Syrah are not from the same grape. They are like parent and child with Petite Syrah being the offspring of Syrah. Adding to the confusion, Petite Syrah is often spelled a variety of ways: "Petit Sirah," "Petite Sirah," or "Petit Syrah." Historically, it has been a product of California winemaking. Petite Syrah is an inky, heavy red wine known for notes of cherry, blueberry, blackberry, plum, smoke, and pepper. Petite Syrah typically does not have a long finish and is often used in blends with other varietals.

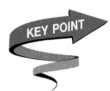 *Syrah and Petite Syrah are not the same grape or wine.*

While Syrah is also known for being dark, it differs from Petite Syrah in that the deep flavor and aftertaste can linger in the mouth. Notes of dark berries, chocolate, espresso, black pepper, and lavender or violet are common. More complex Syrahs can also have secondary hints of tobacco, leather, smoke, and truffle. Other flavors found in Syrah are vanilla, licorice, clove, allspice, rosemary, and mint. Because of the intensity and diversity of Syrah, it pairs well with the heavier dishes associated with barbecue.

The Old World meets the New World with Syrah. The top Syrah producer in the world is France, followed closely by Australia. Old World Syrah from Europe is earthier and more acidic with characteristics of from truffles, florals, smoke, rosemary, minerals, and leather. New World Syrah from the United States and Australia is fruit-forward and "jammier," with heavy spice notes like clove, mint, allspice, licorice, pepper and blueberry.

Wine Regions

Your Passport to the World

Wine is truly the world in a glass (or a bottle). You can experience the far reaches of the planet without having to do the paperwork, deal with airport security, or lug your belongings from place to place. The origins of wine have been traced to the Middle East, but wine has found permanent homes throughout Europe, North America, South America, and Australia. That's not to mention South Africa and a growing wine industry in China.

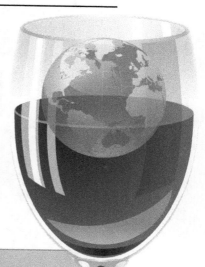

Special Feature...

First Signs of Wine

During an archeological dig in the Zagros Mountains of Iran, 6 clay jars were found in the kitchen area of a Neolithic home dating back to 5400-5000 B.C. One of the jars was big enough to hold 5 liters (2.5 gallons) and had a mysterious yellow film inside it that turned out to be the dried out remains of wine.

Typically, the first place that comes to mind when wine is mentioned is France, but thanks to a seemingly impossible turn of events in 1976, the United States also became a powerhouse in wine. From that breakthrough moment, other regions have enjoyed cultivating wine with great success.

Special Feature...

California Underdogs Win the "Judgement in Paris"

French wines dominated the global market until a May 24, 1976 wine tasting in Paris. Steven Spurrier, an English man with a wine shop in Paris, was introduced to California wines by American students at the nearby L'Academie du Vin. He was curious about how well the California vino would compete against the French heavyweights. Spurrier recruited nine of the best French wine tasters for a blind tasting (meaning they would taste and rate the wines without knowing where they were from until after they had ranked them). The tasting was sold as a celebration of the American bicentennial that the French felt assured would be an easy victory.

Instead of the expected domination, California wines won both the red category and white categories. For the Cabernets, the 1973 Stag's Leap S.L.V. beat the likes of Chateau Mouton-Rothschild and Chateau Haut-Brion. The 1973 Chateau Montelena Chardonnay was rated first over the French Chardonnays of Meursault-Charmes and Puligny-Montrachet among others. The results stunned the French tasters as well as the rest of the world.

Barbara Ensrud from the *Wall Street Journal* called it the wine equivalent of the "shot heard round the world." The 1976 Paris Tasting launched California wine into the same stratosphere as that of the elite French wines. The wine world was never the same.

The movie *Bottle Shock* details the story of Chateau Mantelena's journey to being named the best Chardonnay from the Judgment in Paris.

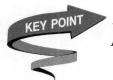

France and California are considered the biggest players in the world of wine.

Other important wine influences abound from places such as Germany, Italy, Spain, Portugal, and throughout Europe. Just as France dominates European wines, California is considered the powerhouse state for American wines, as well as the New World in general. Other regions of the United States, such as Washington State, Oregon, and New York, also have growing wine industries and rising reputations. Wine production has also grown globally, to the point that solid wine finds from Down Under and in places such as Argentina and Chile are no longer surprising.

Special Feature...

While California may be the main force in wines from the Western Hemisphere, the industry's roots in California stem from Europe via Central/South America. As explorers and church padres began to visit and settle in California, they brought wine grapevines from Spain and Italy with them. After all, they needed wine for church services.

The wine industry in California began from the south and moved north as the missions were established up into the West Coast. Wine in California is the result of expansion from south of the border.

France

While most folks use the blanket term "French" to describe wine from France, wine drinkers understand that French wines are products of unique areas within the country's borders. There are roughly 17 wine regions throughout France; of those, the most recognizable are Bordeaux, Burgundy, and Champagne.

Bordeaux

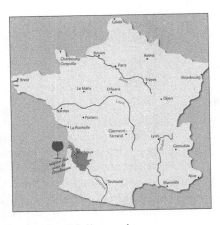

Some of the most famous French wineries are in Bordeaux, including Chateau Mouton-Rothschild and Chateau Haut-Brion. Bordeaux is located in southwestern France near the Atlantic Ocean. About a third of the best quality wines in France comes from Bordeaux, where there are nearly 9,000 wineries and 13,000 grape growers. More than 600 million bottles are produced annually in this region alone, ranging from everyday wine fare to bottles that sell for thousands of dollars each.

The wine produced here is known for the influence of the soil, which is a mix of gravel, clay, and sandy stone. Most of the grapes grown in the region are for the red wine for which the area is known. Although reds dominate regional winemaking, a small percentage (less than 10%) of production includes a few white varietals.

TIP If a wine is referred to as a "Bordeaux" it is typically a mixture of Cabernet Sauvignon, Merlot, and Cabernet Franc (in descending and varying concentrations). With anything generically referred to as a Bordeaux, expect a full-bodied red.

Burgundy

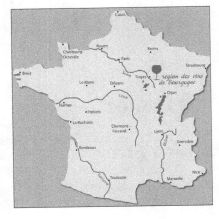

Burgundy is the second French region where the name of the area can be equated to the wine being offered. In Burgundy, the Pinot Noir grape takes center stage. Pinot from Burgundy tends to be focused on earthiness, and winemakers throughout the region constantly reference the wine's terroir. Though White Burgundies do exist, these are less common than reds. White Burgundies regularly use a foundation of Chardonnay, but the Beaujolais district within the area is known for the Gamay grape, while is more popular as a lighter table wine for every day drinking.

Burgundy is southeast of Paris between Dijon and Lyon and includes various districts. The most notable wine areas are the Côte d'Or, which is divided in Côte de Nuits to the north and Côte de Beaune to the south. The area is relatively small, about 12,000 square miles, but it packs more than 5,000 wine growers into the tight quarters. The Côte d'Or is responsible for 90% wine production in the region, so it is truly the epicenter for Burgundy wine.

Author's Aside

I absolutely love the Côte d'Or in the fall, when the vines have turned gold after harvest and the fall foliage is at its peak. The Marche Aux Vins in Beaune (pronounced "Bon") is well worth an afternoon of exploring the caves and tunnels before ending up in the tasting room. Wines cover the full spectrum from table wines to bottles worth thousands of dollars. The more expensive ones are in a locked vault near the exit and are accessed only with special permission. On my second trip there, one of the stewards overheard me talking to my traveling companion. I guess since we sounded knowledgeable enough, we were invited in to the vault just after Brad Pitt and Angelina Jolie left. (If only I had their bank accounts as well.) I left empty-handed from the high-end area but took home a surprise in the form of a 20-year-old, red Burgundy that was economical (roughly $30 versus compared to other bottles in the 5 digit realm). Still, it was fun. Be willing to go on a wine adventure. You never know what opportunities you will get with a little wine knowledge.

Champagne

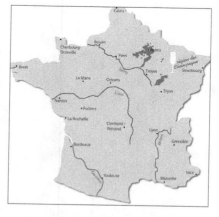

Anyone who has celebrated New Year's Eve knows the major wine product of the Champagne region. The area is located in the northern region in France, east of Paris. The region is unique because of its climate and soil composition. It experiences cool winters and sunny growing and harvest seasons which vines love. Most notably, the soil in Champagne is chalky at the surface which reflects the heat and helps ripen the grapes on the vine even with average temperatures that hover around 50 degrees. Pinot Noir, Chardonnay, and Pinot Meunier are the most grown grapes, which is not surprising given that they are the key grapes in Champagne.

Rhône

In Southern France, the Rhône wine region is named after the river that flows through it. The region is divided in to Northern and Southern Rhône. Wines from the area are typically blends of Syrah with other French varietals and are often referred to as "Rhône wines" or by the name of the appellation d'origine controlee, or AOC from where the wine originates. (That means controlled designation of origin, by the way—it's just a geographical designation the French government uses—hence the acronym. It's their version of an AVA.)

In the Southern Rhône, the most famous AOC is Châteauneuf-du-Pape, while in the northern area the major AOCs are Hermitage and Crozes-Hermitage.

Special Feature...

"Come Quick, I'm Drinking Stars!"

Did you know that Champagne was actually a mistake...or was it? Popular wine mythology credits the invention of Champagne to a 1693 discovery of Dom Pierre Pérignon, a Benedictine monk. The story goes that the monk discovered bubbles in the wine he made. It was due to extra sugars trapped inside that caused a secondary fermentation inside the bottles. He was credited with the creation of Champagne after exclaiming to his brothers in the Abbey, "Come quick, I'm drinking stars!"

The reality, is that the quote and myth may have just been clever marketing stunt by the Abbey in 1821, to increase the prestige of the wines the monks made. Current wine lore attributes the development of sparkling wine to an English scientist named Christopher Merret in the 1662. Merret added sugars to wine to purposely create bubbles, making the growing number of sparkling wine fans in England very happy.

Either way, the stories provide interesting talking points. If you're simply looking for entertainment, it's fun to talk about drinking stars. If you're looking to impress, then mention Mr. Merret for brownie points.

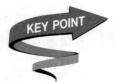

California

California may be considered second to France in regard to wine prestige, but when it comes to influence, the two powerhouses can be seen as equals. Like France, California has numerous winegrowing regions. Wineries and vineyards are found all the way from the North Coast to the Mexican border, and inland along the Sierra Nevada Mountains. The most famous wine regions in California are Napa and Sonoma. Napa Valley is located northeast of San Francisco. The Central Coast of California is also developing a reputation for quality wines. This region extends from Monterey and includes the Paso Robles wine region, halfway between San Francisco and Los Angeles, down to Santa Barbara, with San Luis Obispo and other pockets of vines in between.

Napa

Napa Valley is made up of 16 American Viticulture Areas (AVAs) that have distinct microclimates within the valley. In addition to climate, there are differences in the soil and topographical considerations that impact the wine produced in each AVA. Napa Valley is surrounded by mountains and is the product of both volcanic activity and previous submersion in the ocean. The sediments and geology makes the soil rich and ideal for grape growing. The northern end of the valley is characterized by volcanic influences, which are most noticeable in the soil and the landscape. The southern end of the valley is affected by sedimentary conditions that are evidenced in the resulting wines.

The first commercial vineyard in Napa was established in 1858 by John Patchett. It hasn't always been roses for the wine industry in Napa, or the United States as a whole. California vineyards, like those in Europe, were forced to deal with "Phylloxera Plague" in the 19th century. It infested vines worldwide before California wineries faced the challenges of Prohibition and the Great Depression. Prohibition virtually stopped wine production and consumption in America in the 1920s. When it was repealed, the country faced an economic crisis that caused drinkers to switch to hard alcohol (it was more practical) rather than wine. Napa Valley didn't fully recover until the Judgment in Paris, which put it at the top of the world's wine list.

Special Feature...

The Phylloxera Plague

During the 1860s, grape vines all over France began to wither and die. The Great French Wine Blight, also known as the Phylloxera Plague, began in Britain and spread to France, then throughout the entire European continent. At first, it was a mystery. Some thought it was a curse of some sort. Desperate French winemakers went as far as to bury live toads under vines to draw out the mysterious "poison" killing off the vines.

The answer wasn't toad sacrifices. The reason vines died off was because of Phylloxera, a tiny aphid-like insect. The microscopic sap-suckers fed on the roots and leaves, causing damage that led to fungal infections on the vines that literally sucked the life out of them.

Winegrowers and scientists noticed that vines from Napa Valley were more resistant than European stocks were, but European winegrowers disliked the aromas of the American vines. The answer was the practice of grafting: breeding hybrids that merged the Phylloxera-resistant American stock with the aromas of European vines. To this day, grafting continues to be the preferred method of creating customized and disease-resistant rootstock.

It is estimated that up to 90% of all French vines died in the Phylloxera plague. There is still no "cure" for the problem—winemakers continue the practice of grafting resistant vines to weaker stock.

Napa Valley continues to produce wine associated with some recognizable names: Krug, Staggs Leap, Joseph Phelps, BV, Grgich Hills, Beringer, Hess, Opus One, Robert Mondavi, Screaming Eagle, and Far Niente to name a few. Wines found in Napa run the gamut of varietals grown and wine produced, but Napa Cabernet Sauvignons have the most prominent reputation.

Author's Aside

If you are planning a trip to Napa, the famous, big name wineries are fun to visit, but V Sattui Winery in St. Helena is one of my favorites for an overall enjoyable experience. They offer everything from sweet white wines to robust reds and heavier ports. A tasting option is offered that pairs wine selections with small food platters, too. Warning: it can get extremely crowded because it is a popular stop for organized wine tours as well.

If you like Port wine, don't skip a trip to Prager Winery & Port Works after leaving V Sattui. It's a little hole-in-the-wall tasting room just north of V Sattui on the US-29 behind Sutter Home. Out-of-the-way and cozy are understatements. The ports are to die for, and the pretentiousness of Napa is usually left at the door.

Sonoma

The Sonoma Valley is separated from Napa Valley by the Mayacamas Mountains on the east with the Sonoma Mountains on the west. However, the Sonoma wine region extends all the way to the Pacific Ocean. With 14 AVAs, Sonoma's top varietals, including Chardonnay, Cabernet Sauvignon, Pinot Noir, Merlot, and Zinfandel, reflect the influence of coastal weather as well as the warmer and drier inland conditions.

The history of wine in Sonoma mirrors that of Napa. Franciscan monks planted the first vine in the area at Mission San Francisco Solano in 1823, but the first commercial winery in the Sonoma Valley was Buena Vista Winery, started by Agoston Haraszthy in 1857. Like those in Napa, winemakers in Sonoma struggled with Phylloxera, as well as the cultural, economic, and political challenges of Prohibition and the Great Depression, which were unique to the American wine industry.

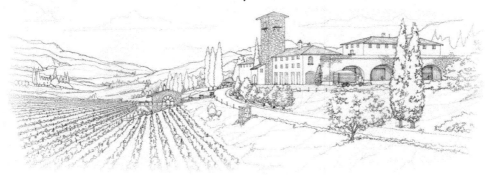

Special Feature...

Depression Follows the Noble Experiment

Nothing jeopardized the American wine industry more than the 18th Amendment to the U.S. Constitution, enacted in 1920. Known as Prohibition or "the Noble Experiment," it outlawed the production, transport, and sale of alcoholic beverages. That means all commercial winemaking was halted from 1920-1933. There were, however, two small loopholes that saved the industry from complete obliteration. First, a small number of wineries were allowed to stay operational in order to make sacramental wine for churches. Second, the head of every household in America was allowed to produce 200 gallons of homemade wine for personal consumption. The California wine industry survived, as well as it could, through producing wine for churches and fulfilling the huge demand for grapes to make into homemade wine.

Due to unfortunate timing, the repeal of Prohibition in 1933 didn't lead to a sudden rebirth of the nation's wine industry. America was in the grips of the Great Depression when the wine industry got the green light to start again, so there wasn't much capital floating around, and anyway, American drinkers had developed a taste for hard liquor.

It wasn't until the 1960s that the American wine industry roused again—just prior to the Paris Judgment that skyrocketed U.S. wines to international fame.

While Napa and Sonoma are distinct wine regions, it is common practice for wineries in either area to use grapes from vineyards in the other region. For example, a Napa winery may produce a Sonoma Zinfandel or a Sonoma Winery may feature a Cabernet Sauvignon with Napa-grown grapes. It really only matters to those who are status-conscious about having an "estate wine."

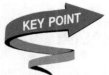

The most notable wine regions in California are Napa and Sonoma.

Central Coast/Paso Robles

The Central Coast of California covers the area south of the San Francisco Bay area at Monterey and extends south along the mountains to Santa Barbara, approximately two hours north of Los Angeles. The most notable wine region in the area is Paso Robles, which was named Wine Region of the Year in 2013 by *Wine Enthusiast* magazine.

Author's Aside

*The Santa Barbara wine region is often the most recognizable wine region in the Central Coast of California, due in large part to its proximity to Los Angeles. It has been featured in various television shows and films. The movie **Sideways** changed the region from a sleepy ranching and wine country community to a destination spot. As a result, wineries in Santa Barbara have become more crowded, expensive, and business-minded. Due in part to its distance from LA, Paso Robles retains some of the more informal wine country ambiance.*

The appellation of Paso Robles is the largest in California, geographically, and also the fastest-growing. It is fourth in the state for the number of acres under vine. The wine region is approximately 25 miles, east to west, and 35 miles, north to south, extending south from the Monterey County to the north to the steep Cuesta Grade near Santa Margarita. The Santa Lucia Mountains to the west buffer the effects of the Pacific Ocean while the Cholame Hills separate it from California's Central Valley.

The area has the most dramatic day-to-night temperature differences of any wine area in California, which aids in the ripening process for vines of all types. More than 45 soil compositions can be found in the Paso Robles region due to marine, volcanic, and seismic influences, which means that soils can vary greatly even within a single plot. The diverse, and in some cases unique, features of the Paso Robles region allow for the cultivation of a full range of distinct wine varieties.

There are currently about 200 wineries operating in Paso Robles.

Wine's Wild, Wild West

Paso Robles is often referred to as the Wild West of California: Jesse James's uncle, Drury James, was the co-founder of El Paso de Robles. After robbing a bank in Russellville, Kentucky in March of 1868, Jesse James and his boys came to Paso Robles and stayed with his uncle, taking advantage of the area's hot springs to heal his lungs from gunshot wounds. Jesse and his men stayed at the La Panza ranch until the end of 1869.

Paso Robles produces a wide variety of wines. The region is known for big, powerful and fruity Zinfandel, and Syrah. Petite Syrah, and a variety of other Italian, French, and Spanish varietals are also grown successfully due to warm temperatures, especially farther inland. Closer to the coast, Pinot Noir vines benefit from cooler conditions.

Other Regions In Europe

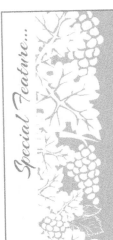

Outside of France, wine drinkers will recognize various areas within Europe that are tied to specific wines. Rieslings are associated with the Rheingau and Mosel areas of Germany, near Frankfurt. The Rheingau is the wine region along the banks of the Rhine River, and the Mosel area is named for the Mosel River, which flows into the Rhine. Italy is most often associated with Chianti wine, named for the region of the same name near Tuscany. Chianti wines are predominantly made from the Sangiovese grape, which is in line with the Merlot, with up to 25% of additional approved varietals added to the mix. Rioja is both a wine region and the wine most associated with Spain. Riojas can be Tintos (reds) or Blancos (whites), with the Tempranillo grape making up approximately 60% of a Rioja Tintos' composition. Portugal and Madeira, a small island off the Portuguese coast, are associated with Port Wines.

Regions in the USA

While California is the most prolific wine producer in the United States, it is not the only state associated with wine production. Nearly all 50 states produce wine. Washington State, Oregon, and New York are the largest producers outside of California, though their combined output equals one-fifth of what California produces each year. Washington is the second largest producer in the United States, with several varietals under cultivation. The most planted varietals in the state are Cabernet Sauvignon, Riesling, Chardonnay, Merlot, and Syrah. The Columbia Valley is Washington's largest wine region and covers approximately 30% of the state. Other areas of note in Washington are the Horse Heaven Hills AVA, with some of Washington's oldest vines, and Yakima Valley AVA, within the Columbia Valley Wine Region, which produces more than 40% of the state's wine. Oregon also shares the Columbia Valley wine region—the Columbia River forms most of its border with Washington. Oregon is known for Pinot Noir, among other varietals. The Willamette Valley is the most recognized AVA in the state.

On the other side of the United States, New York grows many American hybrid varietals, with Vitis Vinifera vines (the traditional wine grape) making up less than 10% of the vines cultivated. The American-French hybrid, Vignoles, is known for producing late harvest and ice wines, though the highest quality New York wines are Rieslings. The Finger Lakes AVA in New York is also known for Chardonnay crafted in a style similar to white Burgundies.

Australian Regions

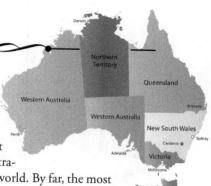

Australia has emerged as a major player in the wine industry, though some critics still dismiss Australian products as "critter wines" because of the popular marketing tactics using animals on wine labels. That doesn't hurt Australia's feelings (or it shouldn't)—Australia is the fourth largest exporter of wine in the world. By far, the most commercially recognized Australian varietal is Shiraz, which is Aussie-speak for Syrah. Other popular varietals grown in Australia include: Cabernet Sauvignon, Merlot, Chardonnay, and Sauvignon Blanc. The Barossa Valley in South Australia is the largest producer in the country. Other areas of note are the Yarra Valley in Victoria and the Hunter Valley in New South Wales. Western Australia's Great Southern, Margaret River, and Swan District have the hottest growing conditions in the entire country.

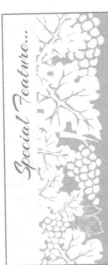

Special Feature...

The Oldest of the Old Vines

Australia's Barossa Valley is located less than an hour from Adelaide. Due to Australia's isolation from the rest of the world and strict agricultural laws, Phylloxera (the nasty pest the nearly wiped out all vineyards in France and Europe) has not infected the soil in Barossa (yet). As a result, it is believed that the region is home to some of the oldest living vines in the world. Syrah wines from old vines in the region, termed "Old Vine Shiraz," are must-try Australian wines.

South America

South America has two countries with wine reputations recognized worldwide. The Mendoza region of Argentina is known for Malbec wines, made from the varietal of the same name. Malbec has its own unique characteristics but is similar to Zinfandel, making it a great paring with red meat dishes. Cabernet Sauvignon is also an important varietal in the Mendoza region. Patagonia is an up-and-coming wine region in Argentina which is gaining a name for itself with its Pinot Noirs. Chile is recognized for Cabernet Sauvignons that mirror Bordeaux Cabernets, as well wines from the lesser known Carmenere grape.

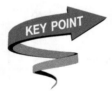

KEY POINT *Other important European regions include the Rhône in France, Germany, Italy, Spain, and Portugal. Oregon, Washington State, and New York are producers in the United States. New World producers include Australia |as well as Argentina and Chile in South America.*

THE TAKEAWAY

We've covered quite a lot in a relatively short time. Now, you have a basic understanding of the types, styles, and core varietals of wine. In addition to learning about the fundamentals, you have also gotten a sense of the world of wine through a quick overview of the world's notable wine regions.

This background will help you understand why wine shops make it a point of labeling distinct areas of the world in relation to the bottles on sale. To quickly review the most notable points from this chapter, use this cheat sheet:

► Wines can be described by type, style, and varietal.

► White wines can be made from either red- or white-colored grapes.

► Rosés are not blended wines made with some white and red wine. They are made by putting the juice in limited contact with grape skins during fermentation.

► The majority of single-varietal bottles do contain a blend of other grapes. The percentage is regulated by the area where the wine is produced. The term "Champagne" should only be used to refer to sparkling wines produced in the French region of Champagne.

► Casks range from large vats to barrels, in which wine fermentation and aging occurs. They are typically made of wood or steel.

► Fortified wines contain the addition of distilled spirits, most often brandy.

► Dessert wines are usually sold in smaller bottles due to cost and sweetness.

► Pinot Gris and Pinot Grigio are from the same grape. Gris is a fuller wine from France, and Grigio is a lighter wine from Italy.

► Chardonnay wines are often characterized by the use of steel or oak during fermentation.

► Any wine can be made into a late-harvest style wine, but Riesling is one of the most commonly used varietals for the dessert wine.

► Syrah is referred to as Shiraz in Australian wines.

► Syrah and Petite Syrah are not the same grape or wine.

► France and California are considered the biggest players in the world of wine.

► The most notable French wine regions include: Bordeaux, Burgundy, and Champagne.

► The most notable wine regions in California are Napa and Sonoma.

► Other important European regions include the Rhône in France, Germany, Italy, Spain, and Portugal. Oregon, Washington State, and New York are producers in the United States. New World producers include Australia as well as Argentina and Chile in South America.

"There is truth in wine, but you never see it listed in the ingredients on the lable."

—Josh Stern

2

Selecting a Bottle

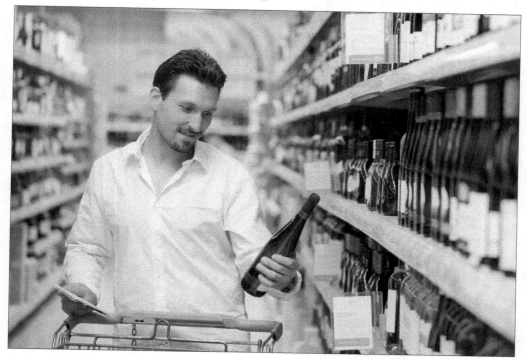

Now that you know about the major wine types and varietals, it is on to the hard part: picking out a bottle to drink. The hundreds of choices you face in the wine aisle of a store can be daunting. Unless you are buying at a winery, you won't get the chance to taste what's inside the bottle before handing over your cash. Buyers have two options: grabbing a random bottle and hoping for the best, or learning a few pointers to help make intelligent selections.

We'll cover the entire process of selecting a bottle of wine. First, an overview of where to buy wine will get you to the right places. Next, we'll cover how to explore the world of wine through your purchases. Then, the discussion will move into the areas of reading a wine label, vintages, and ratings. Finally, other considerations for selecting a wine will tie up the topic of choosing a bottle of wine. By the end of the chapter, you should feel more confident in finding and buying a bottle of wine that you will enjoy.

Where to Buy Wine

Some may laugh. After all, how hard can it be to find a place that sells wine? This is a judgment-free zone, so if you're snickering, remember we are starting at the beginning here. You never know, you might just learn a thing or two anyway. Whether you are going to the grocery store, a specialty wine shop, a winery or wine bar, or browsing the web, here are the basics to help you get a bottle in your hand in no time.

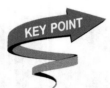

KEY POINT

Wine can be purchased in grocery stores, specialty shops, wineries, wine bars and lounges, and online.

Grocery Stores: Wine on Aisle Nine

Grocery stores and big box retailers are the first places many people start to shop for wine. In some cases, initial wine purchases are at liquor stores or even upscale gas stations. Wine snobs will look down their noses at the mere thought of buying wine at a grocery store because the aisles of a typical store are often populated with wines that are mass produced and lack character. However, the poor reputation of grocery store wines is not necessarily warranted. With a little knowledge, shoppers can locate quality wines and benefit from special savings, too.

Shop Talk...

11. **Grocery Store Wine**, expression. A phrase, usually derogatory, used to describe lower-quality, cheaper wines purchased in grocery stores.

A reference to a bottle being a grocery store wine will often imply that it is lacking in prestige and widely available in restaurants or stores. Wineries produce wines of various qualities, so even more notable names can have an entry level label for sale in grocery stores. Many Australian wines have a reputation for being grocery store wines because of the way they are marketed.

Buying wine at a grocery store does not automatically mean it is poor quality, despite the implication of inferiority by the elitists, however.

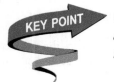

Grocery store wine can have a negative connotation due to mass production and the perception of lower quality.

Buyers will usually be on their own to make their wine selection, as grocery store staff typically do not have specialized training in wine. Once in the wine section, buyers will notice that wines are categorized by type first: reds, whites, sparkling, and Port wines set apart from each other. From there, wines will be grouped by varietal. As a general rule, many red wine sections will follow a similar flow, of lighter style to fuller bodied varietals or vice versa.

For example, the aisle may start with Pinot Noir selections, then Merlot, followed by Zinfandel, Cabernet Sauvignon, and Syrah. This helps the buyer easily locate bottles of specific varietals. If you are looking for a Cabernet Sauvignon, but the first section of reds you encounter are Pinot Noir bottles, you do not have to scan every bottle to know that your Cab is closer to the other end of the red wine section. White wines will often start with Chardonnay wines, simply because that is the most popular white wine purchased. From there, the selections will tend to flow to Pinot Gris/Grigio, then Rieslings and Gewürztraminers.

Once in front of a specific varietal, the wines are not randomly stocked on shelves. There is a logical thought process to grocery store stocking and marketing. The most expensive bottles are placed on the top shelves, unless the store has a special case for expensive wines. The cheapest wines are on the very bottom shelf. The rationale is to encourage the sale of a higher-priced bottle. Wines near the ground stay farther out of the standard line of vision and also require more effort to bend down and retrieve a bottle.

The shelves in between the top and the bottom are where the most competition for wine purchases occur, because this is the area that generates the largest number of sales. This is due to both visibility and a mid-range price point. Wine distributors work hard to stand out in the sea of competitors' bottles. The sweet spot for wine marketing is straight at the standard eye level. Bottles in this area will often be slightly above the mid-range price, but will regularly have sales options that discount prices and encourage purchases.

The overall range in prices at a grocery store can vary dramatically. In higher-end communities or in areas with proven wine consumption, wines on the top shelf can run $60 and up, while the bottom shelf may have bottles for under $5. The selection in more wine-conscious stores will include bottles at that higher end with better reputations, all the way through to the most-recognized labels and cheapest of options. Wine sections in these stores can rival smaller, more specialized wine shops.

In less affluent communities, grocery stores will usually stock the more recognizable, mass-produced labels with price points topping out in the $30 range.

In addition to the wine aisle, shoppers looking for white or sparkling wines that are going to be consumed immediately will want to look in the beer cooler area. Grocery stores often keep a small selection of popular white and sparkling wines chilled so you can take it right home and open it up.

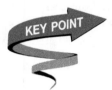

KEY POINT *For white wine and sparkling wine purchases that will be consumed immediately, chilled bottles may be located in the cooler section of the grocery store.*

Grocery stores can provide volume discounts for wine purchases, as well as other special deals to encourage shoppers to buy wines. For example, shoppers might get an extra 10% off of their wines with the purchase of six bottles. Normally, these offers allow for a variety of selections, making it easier to try new wines or stock up on favorites.

Author's Aside

I have no shame in my game when it comes to buying bottles in the wine section of my local grocery store. In fact, it has helped me to avoid having my wine hobby break the bank. I recently saved 40% off of six bottles with some smart shopping—and you can, too, by hunting for deals. Don't avoid the lower shelves of the wine section. On a whim, I picked up a bottle of a Chenin Blanc that was selling for $3 on the bottom shelf. I took it home and actually loved it. The next day, $12 got me six more bottles of it!

In some instances, shoppers will find wine at convenience stores and gas stations. The selection will be limited to the most commercial and mass produced, but if they have a brand you like, go for it. White wines will often be located next to beer in the cooler because people buying wine at a convenience store generally want it chilled for immediate drinking (that's the "convenience" part of "convenience store.") Prices also tend to be higher than in grocery stores because of limited selection and lesser demand.

This is no time to get snobby (there's never a good time to get snobby, actually) about wine at gas stations. On road trips up to Big Sur from Los

Angeles, I always stop at the last gas station in Cambria. Since it is close to Paso Robles, they carry a selection of local wines that I can't typically find elsewhere. On one visit in 2005, I came across a bottle of 1997 Zinfandel among the bottles of 2004s and 2005s. 1997 was a killer year for the wine, and the owner didn't know what he had. I picked up the '97 Zin for a dollar more than the younger wines.

Even outside of wine country, a gas station can yield surprises. While living in Charlotte, North Carolina, I stopped at a local gas station and found a small wine section that included some of my favorite wines from smaller Paso Robles wineries. Who would have thought? They weren't even in the specialized wine shops in the area. Needless to say, that gas station became a regular stop to top off as well as stock up.

Specialty Shops

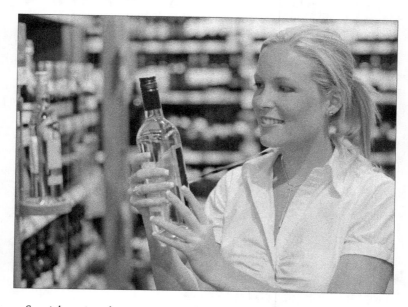

Specialty wine shops can range from large national chains that sell alcohol to liquor stores with an extensive wine selection (often referred to as "Bottle Shops") to small, boutique stores. The major benefits of visiting a specialty wine store rather than a grocery or big box store are that the sales staff is usually knowledgeable about wine and there is often a greater selection.

For specialty shops, the layout differs from most grocery stores, due in part to the larger selection. Reds, whites, sparkling, dessert, and Port wines will still be separated into distinct sections. Within those sections, wines will be delineated by varietal. An additional division is often used to group wines from each country or region of origin. For example, a Pinot Noir section will also have an area for California selections as well as French bottles, and even more specifically for French Pinot Noir—Burgundies.

For the beginner, shopping at a specialty store can be much easier than buying at the grocery store because knowledgeable staff members are available to assist with purchases. In fact, larger retailers keep people on the floor just to help customers make selections. Even if you have no clue about what you want to purchase, they can help you with ideas. They will ask you what you are looking for, or if you have no clue, they'll ask you what you like. By finding out what you already prefer, they can make suggestions about similar wines that you may find enjoyable. Also, shoppers will want to mention the type of situation for which they are buying the wine. If you are looking for a wine to serve with a particular meal, certain wine characteristics are going to be better suited to the food than others.

Specialty stores frequently have special events and sales as well. If you plan to be a frequent wine drinker, it is beneficial to sign up for mailing lists and discount programs. Special events include a variety of wine tastings that can expand your wine knowledge without the expense of buying full bottles. Tastings are usually themed to highlight specific wines. A tasting spotlighting a single varietal, like Chardonnay, will feature wines from different countries and regions. A general tasting will include selections of a range of varietals. Other tastings will highlight a specific style like sparkling wines, ports, or dessert wines. For those learning how to pair food and wine, specialty stores may provide such tastings or at least highlight how to pair food items available in the store with the wine sold. The purpose of the tastings is to sell wine, so be prepared to hear some sales pitches during the event. However, if the tasting isn't free to get in, there is no perceived obligation for you to make a purchase.

Wineries

Wineries offer wines for purchase at their location, online, or through wine clubs. Buying direct is the best option for wine drinkers who are already familiar with specific winery's products. The advantages of purchasing through a winery are a greater selection of that winery's products, regular updates about new offers, and the winery experience when visiting. The major disadvantages include being limited to a single producer's inventory and a lack of convenience in buying wine because of the need to wait for a delivery or to visit the location.

In some cases, the first wine experience a person has is during a tasting trip to wine country. We will discuss wine tasting trips in depth in a later section, but buying wine from a winery can be a way to experience wines that would not be available in stores near home. Buyers have the oppor-

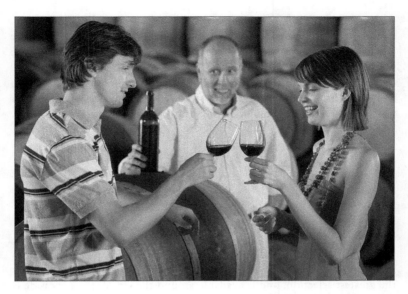

tunity to taste a variety of wines before purchasing as well. The people working in the tasting room have knowledge about the wines for sale in a way that store staff members do not.

Wine clubs give people a chance to build a collection and experience a range of wines. A word of caution: if you are purchasing wines while wine tasting, you may want to refrain from joining wine clubs until you know more about the offerings. Every winery offers a club option to keep sales going, but be careful: It is easy to overextend yourself by joining several clubs on a wine tour—your wallet tends to open a little too fast after a few glasses of wine, so keep your wits about you.

Wine Bars and Wine Lounges

Wine bars and wine lounges are geared more toward selling wine for consumption on the premises, but most will still sell bottles to be taken home. Bottles purchased at a wine bar can be priced at restaurant rates with a steep markup, unless there is a special sale, so you will want to have a sense of pricing before purchasing. If you are interested in buying a wine that you enjoy, you can always make a note and research your buying options later.

Wine bars are an effective way to experience a variety of wines without having to commit to an entire bottle first. Wine bars will have a list of wines—red, white, sparkling, and occasionally ports and dessert wines—at a range of price points. The list will often have a brief description of the wine. If there is no menu, the server will provide you with the available options. Lists will be divided between red and white, and go from lightest

51

to the most full-bodied. In some cases, the sweetest wines will be at the end of a given section. That is because a sweet wine can blow out your taste buds for more subtle wines of a similar type. If you are drinking a variety of wines, it is best to start with the lightest white wine that interests you and work through the list to the most powerful red or dessert wine. That way you will maximize your ability to taste the characteristics of each wine.

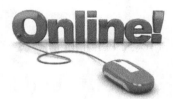

Online

Ordering online, whether through a winery or a major retailer, is an increasingly popular option for buying wine. It is convenient, provides the greatest selection, and is available around the clock. The downside is the lag time between ordering and delivery.

Online wine shoppers need to be aware of the local laws governing wine shipments before buying. Laws vary between states and countries, so shipping wine may not be possible where you live. Wineries can be more limited in shipping options than major retailers due to distribution concerns.

In most cases, an adult over the age of 21 will need to be available to sign for any packages containing wine. Deliveries tend to be done during business hours, so you may need to make alternative arrangements such as delivery to a neighbor's address to sign for the package during the day, delivery to an office instead of your home, or picking up the package at the shipping company's local office.

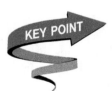

When buying online, wine shoppers need to be aware of the local laws governing wine shipments before buying.

Buyers purchasing wine online can read pertinent information about a given wine such as tasting notes, ratings, pricing, and customer reviews to assist in buying decisions. It is also easier to comparison shop online for better prices. Even if the purchase is not completed online, websites can provide information on wine options and pricing that can assist the buyer with in-store shopping. A general search of wine online can provide a list of wine sellers, and major brick and mortar stores also run online stores.

An additional consideration for online wine purchases is hot weather. Deliveries may be halted if the weather gets too hot because heat damages wine.

Also, wine should not be left outside in the heat during the day, and ideally, wine should be allowed to sit for a day or two prior to drinking to allow for any particles in the wine to settle in the bottle. This is especially important for wines labeled as "unfiltered."

So, now that you know the more popular places and methods for buying wine, we need to get down to the basics of evaluating a bottle of wine.

Bottle Shapes

Wine bottles come in various shapes and sizes. While the size of the bottle is fairly self-explanatory, the reason for the shapes is not as obvious. Some bottles are designed for the specific characteristics of the wine they contain. Other bottle shapes are simply a matter of traditions or novelty. When you get down to it, the shape of the bottle is of relatively little concern to the wine drinker. After all, it's really about what is in the glass.

Instead of discussing the nuances of bottle shapes, this discussion is focused on the absolute basics of bottle shapes, because knowing a general description of the bottles used for different varietals will make the wine aisle easier to navigate.

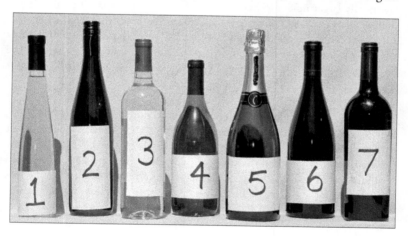

Quick Bottle Rundown

The picture does not show wine bottles in the order that you would serve wine. Instead, the lineup is to make the differences in typical wine bottles more apparent. On the far left, #1 is a bottle of a dessert wine, while bottle #2 is a bottle used for Rieslings and Gewürztraminer wines. Both bottles are more lengthy and narrow. The dessert wine bottle is 375ml compared to the 750 ml Riesling bottle, which is the most common difference for dessert wines. Bottles for Rieslings and Gewürztraminers will also typically be in a darker colored bottle that is brown, green, or even blue.

The more typical bottle shapes are the ones shown in the rest of the picture. The white wines featured in bottles #3 and #4 are ones in which you will find whites such as Pinot Grigio and Chardonnay. Lighter whites are meant to be consumed quickly and not necessarily stored for longer periods, so they will be found in clear or lightly colored bottles. Chardonnays are crafted for both aging and drinking and will be in a shaded bottle that is a deeper gold, green, or even brown. Chardonnay bottles also have more of a bell shape compared to the upright, shouldered bottles of lighter whites.

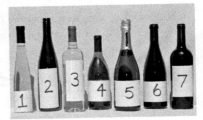

The bell shaped bottle carries over from Chardonnays (#4) to sparkling wines (#5) as well as Pinot Noir (#6). Sparkling wines will have a larger and wider bell shape for the body with a longer neck on the bottle. Another difference between the similar bottle shapes is the bottom. A sparkling wine bottle will have a deeper dimple (or "punt") on the bottom. It's not to cheat drinkers out of bubbly. The purpose of the punt is as a "thumb holder" or where the person pouring the wine places the thumb when handling the bottle from the base while serving as a way to keep the bottle colder longer. Sparkling wine bottles are usually larger in size to make up the difference in volume that the deeper dimple takes away, so you do get the same amount of wine from the bottle. Also, because of the gasses in sparkling wines, the glass for a bottle of bubbly is usually thicker than that of still wines, and the punt acts to strengthen the bottle against the pressure inside. A Pinot Noir bottle will have a shallower punt in the base, while Chardonnay bottles will often have no punt at all.

The final wine shape that you'll commonly find in a store is bottle #7, which is used for Cabernet Sauvignon, Merlot, and many red blends. It is similar in shape to the bottles used for light white wines. These red wine bottles may be wider than the white wine version and have slightly rounded shoulders by comparison. This bottle shape will always be dark for red wines because the bottle is designed to minimize contact with light, which can be damaging to the wine it contains as it ages.

Wine Labels

Wine labels can be both informative and entertaining. These mini billboards on wine bottles have one real purpose: to get a shopper to buy the wine inside the bottle. Wineries spend millions of dollars a year to make sure that they are effective in achieving that goal. Labels are designed with specific markets in mind, from casual wine drinkers to those who have more disposable income to buy at higher price points. The choice of colors, fonts, font sizes, and additional information are all purposefully chosen to draw the buyer's eye and trigger a sale.

Wine Label Marketing... Anything but Random

Due to increases in wine consumption after 2000, the United States is now the number one market in the world for wine, and the primary target for wine imports as well. This makes for stiff competition to get a buyer's attention. It is estimated there are more than 7,558 wineries in the U.S. with many having more than one brand, adding at least another 3,150 wine names. That's over 10,000 brands, without counting wines from other countries.

It is common for wineries overseas to have multiple labels for wines that are sold domestically and internationally. Wineries know that many people buy wine because of the label first and the wine inside second. It is estimated wine bottles have three seconds to "sell themselves" to shoppers before people's attention goes elsewhere.

The label must convey the personality of the winery while also appealing to shoppers across generations. The issue of appeal can be a tricky one. For example, those considered "Baby Boomers" prefer fonts that are easier to read and in larger sizes. Boomers find that dark labels with light colored text are more difficult to read. Conversely, younger "Millennials" are drawn to fun labels with bold colors, eye catching names, and quirky shapes. Wineries are creating new, unique labels all the time, including those made of wood and holograms. Peel away labels allow wineries to offer additional information or a QR code to get buyers to scan for special offers or to offer serving suggestions. Anything that gets a shopper to hold a bottle for more than three seconds is the goal for wine marketers. That's the purpose of the wine label, first and foremost.

Labels help shoppers reach for the bottle of wine initially, but the attention-getting tactic is balanced with the need to cover basic information that will assist the shopper in the purchasing decision. Regardless of font, colors, images, and other marketing ploys, the label on a bottle of wine must cover the "Four Ws." They are the "who," "what," "when," and "where."

"Who" covers the winery that makes the wine. Some wineries may even name the winemaker specifically. "What" is the varietal used in the bottle such as Riesling. In cases where the wine in a blend, the varietal may not be listed on the front label, but the varietals in blends (red or white) are often listed on a back label with additional information and descriptions about the wine. However, blends that are expected in wine, such as Bordeaux or Rhone wines, will not typically list the varietals used. "When" is covered with the year, also known as vintage, listed on the bottle. The "where" can be as broad as a country, state, wine region, or a specific vineyard. Occasionally, an additional "how" is part of the wine label for circumstances like different fermentation processes or other relative information. A Chardonnay label may include information about oak or steel being used in the winemaking process, or a Riesling may be defined as a late harvest to orient the buyer better on what to expect from the wine in the bottle.

French wines have traditionally been labeled by Appellation rather than varietal. For example, a bottle will be labeled "Beaune" rather than Pinot Noir. The trend is starting to change though with more European winemakers adopting varietal labeling.

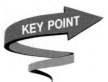

French wines are often labeled with the appellation (geographic origin) rather than the varietal contained in the wine.

It is easier to understand wine labels when you can see one. You will see two simplified wine labels on the following page to help you practice reading a label. There are no pretty pictures or crazy fonts. (After all, I'm not trying to sell you wine.) However, the examples provide a stripped-down view of the information you need to know from a wine label.

A version of an American wine label is the first example, with a French label sample to follow.

Reading an American Wine Label

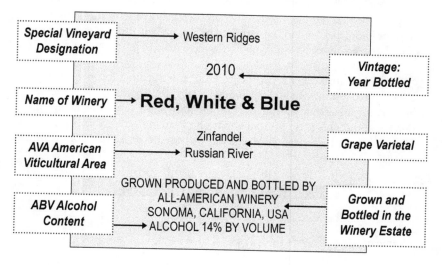

Now you can see how the four Ws (who, the what, when, and where) are depicted on a typical American wine label. This is not representative of every piece of information a label may show. For example, an alcohol warning about drinking while pregnant, the volume of the bottle (i.e. 375 ml), or any preservatives in the wine may be present on the label. Of course, it's also usually done in a more eye-catching manner as well. The labels for French wines, and all imports for that matter, vary slightly as to the core information depicted.

Reading a French Wine Label

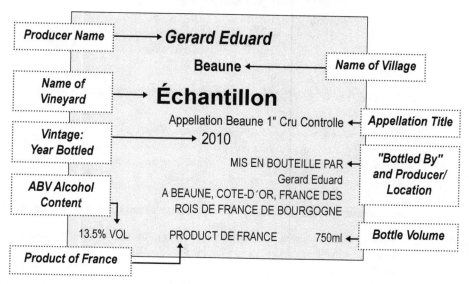

In addition to the Four Ws, imported wines will have a clear "Product of…" statement as well as identifiers for the producer and location. Though not listed here, the domestic importer, in most cases, will also be named on either the front or back label, so don't be surprised by a seemingly obscure reference to a place like New Jersey on your imported wine bottle.

Back labels are a way for wineries to keep your attention for more than the critical three-second window to promote a sale. The additional label provides both required information not listed on the front and a supplemental description about the wine to tip your purchasing decision in that specific wine's favor. With the example of a back label, you can see how the "sales pitch" for the wine is further developed.

Example of a Back Label

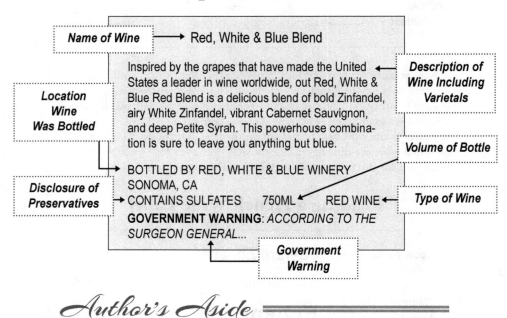

Author's Aside

Yes, before some readers grind their teeth at the mention of White Zinfandel, this is a made up wine. I can't say that White Zinfandel is never part of a red blend for sure, but I haven't seen one. I don't think anyone has thought to even do that. It's just a little wine humor.

It really is that simple. The information needed to understand a wine label is easy to find when you remember to look for the four Ws. Laws dictate that certain information must be included on wine labels to inform the public properly about certain concerns. For wines from overseas, there may be some language considerations that could make understanding a label a little more challenging. If you shop where staff can help you understand the more unique terms to a particular country's wine (such as classes of German Rieslings), you should be able to get help and be able to shop on your own in no time.

Vintages

Vintage is a word thrown around by wine drinkers that can make those new to wine a bit nervous, though it really is a simple concept. It refers to the year the grapes were picked from the vines.

Shop Talk...

> 12. **Vintage**, noun. The year in which grapes used in a wine are harvested. To be clear, it is not the year the vines were planted. It is the year the grapes were picked for processing.

Vintages are listed as a year on most bottles of still wines and single year blends. For example, a bottle of Cabernet Sauvignon will have "2012" on the label to tell the wine drinker that all the grapes in that wine came from the 2012 harvest. A blend that uses grapes from a single season may also have a vintage listed though it uses multiple varietals.

There are exceptions to the rule on vintage labeling. Cheaper, branded wines will not always have vintages listed on them. Champagne and Port wines also do not tend to have vintages on them, but not because of quality. For these styles of wine, it is common for grapes from multiple vintages to be used to create a recognizable "house style" that makes the wine distinctive. In these cases, vintage bottles are only produced when a given year produces outstanding grapes that allow for a single year's grapes to make up the total lot of wine. The vintage classification in the case of Port wines can take years to determine. Port wine is aged in oak barrels for two years before the quality of the wine is assessed for vintage classification. Due to this strict adherence to quality assessment, there are typically only a few vintage years of Ports or Champagnes in any given decade.

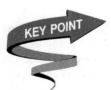

Vintage refers to the year that the grapes used in a wine were harvested. Vintage bottles will lag two or more years due to aging before sale.

Why is vintage important? After all, a Zinfandel vine produces the same types of grapes year after year, right? Well, no, actually they do not. Wine is a product of many factors including everything from Mother Nature to the winemaker tinkering with juice combinations to highlight the characteristics of each year's wine production. Nature plays the first and often most critical role in the resulting wine from any given harvest. Each vineyard is part of a microclimate that influences the vines from budding (when grapes first appear) to ripening.

Shop Talk...

13. **Microclimate**, noun. A microclimate is a distinct geographic area that has different atmospheric conditions from surrounding areas. A microclimate can be identified with a matter of feet, making it possible to have more than one microclimate in a single vineyard.

The distinctions that make up a microclimate include temperature differences and humidity or moisture levels. An area situated near urban areas can have higher temperatures and conversely, areas near bodies of water can be impacted by cooling influences. Also, the slope of the land parcel can impact the microclimate where south-facing slopes in the Northern Hemisphere are exposed to more direct sunlight for longer periods of time each day, resulting in warmer conditions. The opposite is true for the Southern Hemisphere where north-facing slopes receive more direct sunlight. This is important in vineyards because varietals have different optimal growing climates. For example, a Syrah vine thrives in hotter and dryer conditions while a Pinot Noir vine needs to be in an environment with substantial nighttime cooling to produce the best grapes.

Larger climate issues can also impact a vintage. Cold and rain can cause grapes to not ripen properly. A late spring cold snap can prevent grapes from budding until later in the season, shortening the growing period. The result could be under-ripened grapes at harvest time, which produce a wine that is lower in quality. Rainy weather can also "water down" wine produced in a given year because vines are sensitive to the amount of water they receive and a lack of sunlight stops grapes from developing the adequate levels of sugar for a higher quality wine.

On the other hand, dry weather can also affect the wine produced in any given year. When vines are subjected to long periods of hot sunny weather early in the season, budding can happen earlier. With more direct exposure to sunlight, grapes tend to ripen faster. If grapes are allowed to over-ripen, it changes the sugar concentrations in the wine produced. The result is that wine will skew towards more of a jammy taste. For those who prefer big fruit in their wine, it may not be a bad thing, but those who prefer more subtle wines view it is a problem. Drought conditions can also mean that vineyard yields are smaller, meaning that the amount of wine produced in a dry season is less than in other years.

TIP When looking for wine, the vintage listed will typically lag by two years or more because wine needs to be aged to develop its full flavor. Red wines need to sit in oak for years to develop many of their characteristic tastes. Whites, especially those aged in steel, tend to be aged for shorter periods of time, but it is still common to see Chardonnays aged for at least two years in oak before being released.

Entire vintages can be rated just as single wines are. Based on conditions and the historical background of wines from a given region, wine experts will sample a collection of wines from a year's harvest in a particular area and determine a score that reflects the quality of wine produced in that entire region for the given year. The rating of a vintage is an overall trend. It does not guarantee that all wines produced in the region are as good or as bad as the rating indicates. Think of it as the average for wines in the area for that particular year.

A vintage rating is a broader yardstick than an individual wine rating. When using vintages for buying decisions, you need to know more than a blanket claim such as "2005 was an outstanding year." Yes, some areas of Bordeaux and Burgundy had exceptional wines that year, but picking a 2005 Zinfandel from Northern California could lead to a disappointing "average" experience. If you are using the rating of the vintage to select wine, be sure you know the specifics for the region and varietal that you are targeting. Vintages are not a world-wide thing like many new to wine believe.

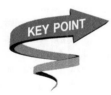 **KEY POINT** *A vintage rating is a broader yardstick than an individual wine rating for determining the likely quality of a bottle of wine.*

Beaujolais Thursday

The exception to the "aging rule" for wine releases by vintage is Beaujolais Nouveau (pronounced [Bo-zho-lay New-vo]). Think of it as Black Friday for the wine community. On the third Thursday in November, wine drinkers flock to wine shops to celebrate "Beaujolais Nouveau Day." The Beaujolais wines are "new" wines, meaning that they are fermented just a few weeks before being released. The wine is from the Gamay grape grown in Beaujolais, France in the Burgundy wine region. Winemakers rush to get bottles of the Beaujolais Nouveau shipped worldwide, which go on sale at 12:01am on the third Thursday in November.

Until World War II, winemakers in Beaujolais released the year's newest wine locally to celebrate the harvest. When the Beaujolais AOC was officially created in the late 1930s, laws were enacted to prevent the sale of the celebration wine before December 15th of the harvest year. In 1951, the rules were relaxed and "Beaujolais Nouveau Day" was created. Call it a nod to tradition or a shrewd marketing stunt, but "Beaujolais Nouveau Day" has winemakers in the region scrambling to have the first bottles of a vintage on the market, around the world, every year. It's profitable for them and an excuse to raise a glass to another year of wine for the rest of us.

Ratings

This brings us to what is probably the most baffling element in wine selection: wine ratings. Wine lovers can be found who claim to drink only "90 point wines" or jump at the chance to taste a 100 point wine. The snobs will look down their nose if they find you with a glass of a wine rated at a mere 85 points. This isn't some innate characteristic of the wine. This is all about the evaluation of the wine in comparison with other vintages and what the varietal is supposed to taste like ideally. First and foremost, like with any type of criticism (wine, books, art, film, etc.), it is in large part subjective with a nod to some objective elements. If you find that you love a given wine that happens to be 85 points, so be it. Ratings are a guidepost, not a hard, fast rule.

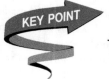

Ratings are not universal to all wines of a given year. A good year for one varietal in one region may not be good everywhere.

When it comes to wine ratings—like the saying about opinions and certain, um, bodily orifices—everyone's got one. Each person has a way of rating the wines they like. Experts and professionals abound with evaluations of wine quality, but there are a few big names that stand apart from the crowd. Robert M. Parker, Jr. is likely the most recognized name and the wine critic with the most weight in wine circles. If you spend any time around wine culture, you are guaranteed to see or to hear mention of his name.

Parker is credited with instituting the 100-point rating system for wine ratings. Until the 1970s, ratings were usually given by those who had ties to the wines being reviewed, either as a producer or seller. In other words, the winemaker or the person selling the wine would create the reviews for the product. Parker recognized this as a conflict of interest. It was a problem for the wine drinkers who were looking for good value in their wine selections. The then-lawyer created *The Baltimore-Washington Wine Advocate* newsletter in 1978 as a way of helping wine buyers get objective information about wines. He devised a scale of 50-100 points based on a wine's aroma and bouquet, appearance and color, flavor and finish, and overall quality or potential for aging.

The 100-point scale created by Robert Parker, and imitated by many others, breaks down as follows:

96—100 = Extraordinary
  (these are the ones to remember and write home about)
90—95 = Outstanding
  (these will put a smile on your face and have you doing a little dance)
80—89 = Above Average to Excellent
  (these are wines that will not leave you completely disappointed but won't necessarily have you jumping either)
70—79 = Average
  (these are the ho-hum "at least it's wine" types of experiences)
60—69 = Below Average
  (these are the ones that you hope that you didn't spend any money on)
59 and Below = Appalling
  (these are the ones you just simply spit out and go to something else)

Nobody likes a critic—unless they say something nice about you, and even critics are subjected to other critics. While Robert Parker and *Wine Advocate* have become a benchmark in wine ratings, there are still some factions in the wine world who view Parker and his wine ratings with some degree of skepticism. The notion of a "Parkerization" of wine has sprung up; some in the community claim that Parker has a preference for riper, less acidic wines that are heavy in oak and alcohol. As a result, it seems that wines have been made to suit his particular tastes in order to get better ratings. However, the shift in winemaking may not be because of Parker's personal preferences. Since the early 1980s, wine growers have been allowing grapes to mature longer on the vine thanks to Émile Paynaud. He is called the father of "International Wines" because of his influence in changing the way wine was made in the late 20th century. This shift is what is referred to not only as the "International Style" of wine but also negatively associated with "Parkerization."

Parker, himself, has addressed the subjective nature of wine ratings by admitting that a scoring difference of a couple of points within a category (for example between 97 and 99 points) could be attributed to something as random as his mood at the time of the evaluation. Parker states that there can never be a substitute for your own tasting experience because the rating is merely one person's assessment of a wine in relation to its peers.

Still, he holds enough clout that an entire vintage can be forced down in price at the hint of a poor assessment. Some go to extraordinary lengths to dispute poor reviews, including death threats. In one case, a French winemaker was so outraged at a negative review that he invited Parker back to the estate to taste again. When Parker arrived at the winery, the manager's dog bit Parker's leg. When Parker asked for a bandage, the manager simply threw him a copy of the bad review. Ouch!

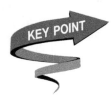 *Ratings are subjective, based on a critic's tastes.*

Robert M. Parker, Jr. and his *Wine Advocate* may be the most recognized wine ratings in the industry, but they are not the only ones. Other wine ratings of note include *Wine Spectator and Wine Enthusiast*. Both of these popular magazines in the wine industry have a solid reputation for their ratings and are referred to frequently in wine shop shelf cards and wine-related media. While browsing for wine in larger retailers or specialty boutiques, buyers may also note the store will post in-house reviews of wine done by staff members or owners. As with all wine ratings, the real vote comes down to your personal tastes. The ratings can help you gauge the likelihood that you will find a particular wine pleasing. Only you have your unique taste buds and preferences, so ratings are not the end-all be-all of making a successful wine selection.

Shop Talk...

14. **Cult Wine**, noun. A wine that is distinguished by stellar reviews, low production, a famous winemaker, and sales usually done through mailing lists rather than through retailers. Most typically associated with Bordeaux-like California reds featuring Cabernet Sauvignon, Cabernet Franc, and Merlot. Some of the more notable cult wines are associated with wineries such as Screaming Eagle, Opus One, Harlan, and Colgin.

Special Feature...

Cult Wines

In the wine community, the term "**cult wine**" is thrown around from time to time. These wines end up being big names because of branding and quality, reflected in the elusive 100-point rating. There are no hard and fast rules about what makes a wine become a cult wine. Though specific wines have been prized throughout history, cult wines burst onto the wine scene in the 1990s as wines got bigger, bolder, and featured longer finishes. These wines were viewed as catering to Robert Parker's tastes and received top scores. The cult wine craze was born in California through a combination of high scoring wines and a booming economy in the 1990s and early 2000s that helped drive prices through the roof. The wines became viewed as trophies, as well as investments, by collectors.

Unfortunately, the cult craze fizzled dramatically with the economic downturn in 2008. Bottles of cult wines that once debuted for between $150 and $500 and soon climbed in value to the $1,000-$2,000 range stopped selling.

Critics of cult wines often cite the elitist nature of selling only to tightly controlled mailing lists as a detrimental practice in the wine industry. Others believe that California's cult wines have no real history (unlike Burgundy or Bordeaux wines), so they are simply a function of a 100 point rating.

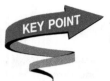

Robert Parker is the most recognizable wine critic/wine rating, but other experts do exist.

Other Considerations When Selecting a Wine

We've covered the basics: where to buy wine, reading a wine label, wine vintages, and wine ratings. There are other factors that can impact a shopper's selection of a wine, including whether a wine is unfiltered or organic. In some cases, the size and shape of a wine bottle is part of the decision to purchase a wine. Also, the fact is that buyers often pick wine to give as gifts for a full range of occasions, from a backyard get-together to a major life event. For that reason, we are going to cover some of the additional elements that can influence the selection of a wine.

Unfiltered Wine

Most mass-produced wines are processed through a very fine filter to remove any lingering particles that can make the wine appear cloudy. In some cases, usually with smaller "boutique" wineries, the wine is not put through the finest of filters, allowing small amounts of sediment to flow into the bottle with the wine. Though there is some degree of filtering, the term for these wines is "unfiltered". Some believe the residual matter adds to the complexity of the wine. The sediment is not a danger, but it is also not very pleasant tasting. For that reason, care should be taken when pouring an unfiltered wine to reduce the amount of sediment that enters the glass.

Shop Talk...

15. **Unfiltered**, adjective. Unfiltered is used to describe wine that is not run through the finest-pored filters typically used in winemaking. The result of an unfiltered wine is that tiny particles can be in the bottle resting at either the bottom or side of the bottle until poured.

There can be a slight grittiness on the tongue with an unfiltered wine, even after steps are taken to minimize the amount of particulates that make it to the glass. In some cases, drinkers may notice a slight buildup on their teeth and tongue from the material. The tannins and aroma can vary slightly between an unfiltered and filtered wine because of the remaining bits of grape skins which make up the particles. Most noticeably, the clarity of the wine will be lessened if an unfiltered wine is jostled. The result is a cloudy appearance that sometimes remains even after the wine has rested and settled in the glass.

Unfiltered wines should be decanted before pouring into glasses in order to allow the wine to open up and the particles to settle before sipping. (We will be discussing more on decanters and letting wines open up in the coming sections.) Unfiltered wines are for the more patient wine drinker who has time to let things settle before popping the cork and letting the wine flow. Let's just suffice it to say that unfiltered wines should not be opened immediately, unless you like the grit in your experience.

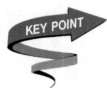

KEY POINT

Unfiltered wines contain more particles in the wine that are believed to add to the complexity of flavor.

Organic Wine

An organic wine has to adhere to the same USDA and National Organic Program (NOP) guidelines—such as restrictions on the use of fertilizers, pesticides, and herbicides—as other food and beverages that are labeled as organic. The difference with wine is the added regulations regarding the addition of **sulfites** in a wine labeled as organic.

Shop Talk...

16. **Sulfites**, noun. Sulfites are a form of sulfur used as a preservative because wine is unstable (meaning quick to break down and turn bad).

The practice of adding sulfur to wine dates back to Roman times as a way to stopping wine from turning into vinegar. In the 20th century, sulfur was found to stop yeasts and bacteria from growing as well as enhancing the red in wine color. Some believe that sulfites are one of the reasons for migraines when drinking wine. Approximately 10% of people with asthma also have a severe sulfite sensitivity, which led to labeling requirements for sulfites in the United States and Australia.

Organic wines must display the USDA organic seal and give information about the agency that certified that the grapes were grown organically. There are four categories that wines complying with organic laws can claim: "100% Organic," "Organic," "Made with Organic Ingredients," and "Some Organic

Ingredients Included." Each designation is tied to the thoroughness in which the organic process is followed throughout winemaking.

Any wine, organic or not, can have naturally occurring sulfites. Those with a sulfite level of more than 10 parts per million must be labeled as "containing sulfites." An organic wine cannot have any **added sulfites**. If there are no added sulfites, the organic wine can be labeled as "Sulfite Free" or "No Added Sulfites-Contains Naturally Occurring Sulfites" where appropriate.

The number of wineries with organic wine lines continues to grow. Notable names such as Domaine Carneros, Grgich Hills, DeLoach Vineyards, and Frog's Leap in California have organic wine selections. Badger Mountain Vineyard and Snoqualmie Wines and Badger Mountain Vineyard in Washington State also do organic wines. Overseas, numerous wineries in France, Australia, and New Zealand are producing organic wines, as are Nova Cappelletta in Italy, Bodega Hermanos Delgado in Spain, and Yarden in Israel.

Locating organic wine is getting easier thanks to specialty grocery stores like Whole Foods emphasizing organic selections, and larger retailers creating shelf space for designated organic wines. Also, online wine sellers will often have a special tag for wines in this category.

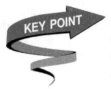

KEY POINT

Organic wines are readily available and are made under strict standards to eliminate or minimize the presence of various chemicals and sulfites.

Bottle Sizes

Like the wine label, the bottle a wine comes in can be a function of volume, tradition, creative marketing, or a combination of them all. Let's start with the more common sizes that wine shoppers encounter. The "standard" bottle is the most recognizable size, obviously. It is the most commonly used size for distributors of wine with a volume of 750 ml. That equals about five standard glass servings. The "piccolo," "split," or "half bottle" is just that, about half the size of a standard at 750 ml a bottle. Half bottles are common with dessert wines, especially ice wines, and expensive wines where the winery wants to provide a low price point option for consumers. At the other end of the standard spectrum is the "magnum" which is 1.5 liters and the equivalent of two standard bottles.

The "double magnum" is the next step up in bottle size for wine. It is 3 liters in volume and equals two magnums or four standard bottles. Boxed wine is often sold in the double magnum size.

Box Wine

We arrive at what is probably the most accepted form of wine snobbery: box wine. Box wine is also known as "cask wine." In the mid-1960s, an Australian named Thomas Angove patented the wine box, which consisted of a plastic bladder holding wine that was encased in cardboard. Despite a less than stellar reputation as a "cheap wine," box wine does have some advantages. The packaging is cheaper and easier for shipping compared to bottles, and now there is an association with boxed wine being more environmentally friendly. Oxidation, which taints and deteriorates wine once it makes contact with air, is minimized if not prevented because of the seal and bladder in the box.

Boxed wines are meant for immediate consumption rather than long-term storage. The wines typically found in boxed format are associated with mass-produced, lower quality and cheaper wines, though midlevel wineries have experimented with box wine selections. Boxed wine can be found throughout the world from Australia to Europe to the United States. With that being said, the wine community tends to look down its nose on the box wine cousins of bottled wine. The long-standing tradition has been that wine is kept in bottles. Like those who deviate from any tradition, boxed wine faces a backlash from the community in the form of a lesser reputation.

Other Bottle Sizes

Now, the talk of bottle sizes reaches the level of crazy, if you are focused solely on drinking and not aging. Bottle sizes larger than a double magnum are normally associated with long-term cellaring rather than party drinking, unless you are a king that is. Large-format wine bottles are named with royal references, many of which church-going folks will recognize. More than likely though, you'll be hard-pressed to get a look at wine bottles at these sizes except for maybe the Imperial and its sparkling wine counterpart. They surface from time to time at major events, if you're lucky.

At this size, there is a distinction between bottles used for still wines and sparkling wines. The thought is that the added pressure of the gases in sparkling wine necessitates a more bell shaped bottle to avoid explosions compared to what bottles for still wine can handle. A "Jeroboam" contains 4.5 liters of still wine. The same sized bottle of sparkling wine is called a "Rehoboam" and is equal to six standard bottles in one. Talk about my kind of six-pack! The 6 liter "Imperial" is equal to two Double Magnums or eight standard bottles of still wine. The same size bottle for sparkling wine is called a "Methuselah." Now we are talking! 40 glasses of wine in a single bottle!

At this point, wine bottle sizes are more about answers on Jeopardy than the wines you will encounter. However, to be thorough, a Salamanzar is 9 liters in volume and holds an entire case of wine in a single bottle. The Balthazar is 12 liters and the equivalent of 16 standard bottles, while the king of them all, a Nebuchadnezzar, holds a whopping 15 liters of wine. That's 20 standard bottles, or 100 glasses of wine. Good luck hoisting that one.

Selecting Wine as Gifts

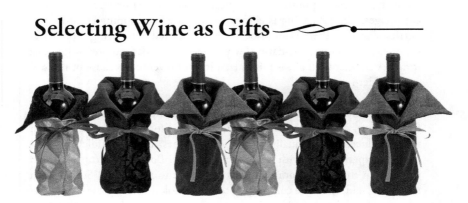

If you are selecting a bottle of wine as a gift or you are simply bringing a bottle to avoid being empty handed at the next backyard get-together, some basic pointers can assure that you don't bring something that is destined to turn to vinegar before anyone dares to drink it. Gifting wine is easiest for those whose wine preferences you already know, even if it is just which type of wine they enjoy most. Paying attention to what people drink before giving a bottle of wine gives you an idea of what to target, be it the same bottle or a similar one. In those situations, you can choose to get what the person already drinks, or decide to give them a similar bottle for them to explore. For example, if the person enjoys California Syrah from a specific winery with their barbecue, you may go with a Syrah from the same winery. Instead, you may decide to give a California Syrah from a different winery or go in a different direction with an Australian Shiraz to compare their favorite to, as a way to help them branch out a little.

Those are the simplest decisions when gifting wine, but what if you have no idea what the person likes when it comes to wine? If you're not even sure that the person is a wine drinker, it is best to stick to traditional varietals. In these cases, a Chardonnay as a white wine is a safe bet. For those looking for an easy grab and a popular option which is widely available, Kendall-Jackson Chardonnay is a good option around $12 a bottle. A slightly elevated option that has a good balance of oak and fruit is the Chardonnais Chardonnay from Napa Valley. It retails for between $20 and $30.

Finding a red wine gift option for those who are new to wine can be a bit trickier. Many people who are new to wine talk about not liking "dry" wines when they mean that they prefer sweet wines. The term dry is often wrongly associated with a perception of alcohol burn and heavier wines which need to be consumed with food to be fully appreciated. Those who are not familiar with wine tend not to like wine with more tannins because they are less "drink-on-their-own" friendly. Those who prefer a bottle to sip rather than one with a full meal will find a red blend more pleasing. A personal favorite of mine, which is widely available in stores, is the Apothic Red Blend. It has a mix of the big four red varietals with Cabernet Sauvignon, Zinfandel, Syrah, and Merlot and is a touch on the sweeter side, making it a good sipping wine as well as a solid pair for many foods. It is relatively budget friendly at around $10-12 a bottle and widely available in stores.

Author's Aside

Apothic red became my go-to "Tuesday Night Spaghetti Wine" after a spur of the moment selection on a store run. It has a friendly price point and is my kind of wine for a weekday dinner or a simple glass to celebrate the end of the workday. Since then, it has proven to be a favorite with my friends as a solid gift wine too. Apothic does an approachable wine blend as well that is well-balanced and includes Chardonnay, Riesling, and Moscato, at around the same price as the red.

Now that I've given you an insight, just be sure not to buy it all up and make it hard for me to find. Otherwise, my weeknights will be a lot less jovial.

If you are bringing a bottle of wine for a specific situation, like a Christmas dinner or barbecue, other gift options are appropriate as well. For a barbecue, a fruity California Zinfandel or a bold Syrah work well with grilled red meats. For Christmas dinner with a ham centerpiece, a Riesling works well with the saltiness of the ham, as does a Pinot Noir or a Rosé. Thanksgiving dinner and turkey match well with Rieslings, Gewürztraminer, Pinot Noir, and Zinfandel.

Screw Top Wine

Like box wine, screw top wine has the connotation of being cheap wine. This is not really the case. More wineries are experimenting with screw tops and other synthetic corking materials for several reasons. Corks are prone to spoiling and can cause wine to go bad. Screw tops can avoid the potential of a bottle going south before it can be enjoyed. Also, cork is a natural product of the cork tree, which has been repeatedly overharvested. When cork supplies run low, wineries look for other more economical and effective ways to cap their bottles. A growing number of wineries are using synthetic corks as a result. Whether it is a natural cork, a synthetic cork, or a screw top, it is really about the wine inside the bottle, not the way it is capped. Wine snobs may look down their nose since tradition dictates a natural cork, but the reality is, as long as the wine is sealed against oxygen and doesn't leak, it is about what goes in the glass, not what is at the top of the bottle.

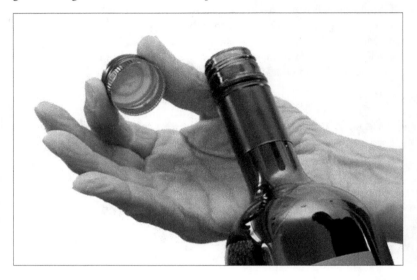

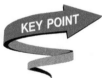 *Boxed and screw topped wines may be perceived as inferior, but both have benefits that protect wines against damage.*

THE TAKEAWAY

While finding a place to purchase wine is easier than ever, it can feel like you need a decoder ring to figure out how to select bottles when you first begin to explore wine. Now you know all about the ways in which you can select a bottle without having to play "eeny-meeny-miny-moe" and simply hoping for the best. To recap:

▶ Wine can be purchased in grocery stores, specialty shops, wineries, wine bars and lounges, and online.

▶ Grocery store wine can have a negative connotation associated with it because of mass production and the perception of lower quality.

▶ For white and sparkling wine purchases that will be consumed immediately, chilled bottles may be located in the cooler section of the grocery store.

▶ For online wine purchases, buyers should be aware of local laws governing the shipment of alcoholic beverages.

▶ French wines are often labeled with the appellation (geographic origin) rather than the varietal contained in the wine.

▶ Vintage refers to the year that the grapes used in a wine were harvested. Vintage bottles will lag two or more years before sale due to aging.

▶ Ratings are not universal to all wines of a given year. A good year for one varietal in one region may not be good everywhere.

▶ Ratings are subjective, based on a critic's tastes.

▶ Robert Parker is the most recognizable wine critic/ wine rating, but other experts do exist.

▶ Unfiltered wines contain more particles in the wine that are believed to add to the complexity of flavor.

▶ Organic wines are readily available and are made under strict standards to eliminate or minimize the presence of various chemicals and sulfites.

▶ Boxed and screw topped wines may be perceived as inferior, but both have benefits that protect wines against damage.

"I cook with wine;
sometimes I even add it to the food."

—W. C. Fields

$\mathcal{3}$

Basic Food & Wine Pairings

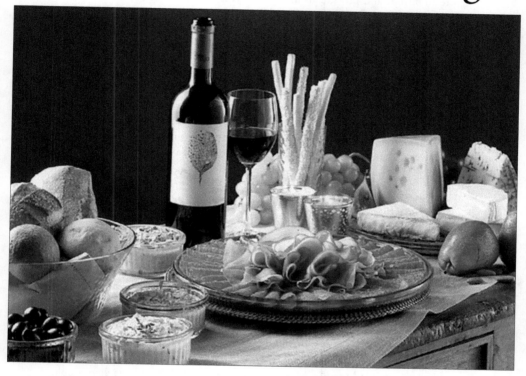

Food and wine are truly meant to go together. Sure, there are wines that make for good solo sipping, but to get the full flavor of a wine, and to counter some of that tipsy toasting, food is as important as the wine itself. If you are looking for a quick answer to the perfect food to go with all wine, you're out of luck. The best answer in that case is simply: eat and drink what you like. Not very helpful, right? What can I say? The reality is that certain wines will "pop" with foods that enhance their flavors.

After reviewing the varietals, it should be obvious that each wine has a unique character. Food also has its own personality. Asian foods can be spicy in a way that is different from Mexican food. A good burger or steak calls for a wine that is different than one for a salad. Even the ubiquitous wine and cheese pairing is not as cut and dry as one would initially think. It can be a fun food adventure to explore how wine and food work together, if you have the time and money to do so.

continued...

However, not everyone does. As a result, this section will provide some simple pointers for food and wine pairings that cover everything from party or picnic nibbles to special dinners.

The process of pairing food and wine can start with a specific dish for which you need to find a wine match, or the wine can be used to decide the food menu. Some matches are made in heaven (kind of like a culinary soul mate relationship) and provide an unexpected zing, while others are like comfortable and reliable best friends to each other. Some pairings are seen as ideal or standard fare. However, if you do not like a certain food, like lamb for example, even a perfect wine probably won't make the meal more enjoyable.

To try to make some sense of the millions of possibilities for food and wine pairings, this section will be divided in two ways. The first section will focus on cheeses and wines with an emphasis on pairings that work well for nibbles and party favors, since wine is often a social event. The second section will focus on matching varietals with specific meals and food dishes. Consider the first section the "appetizer" for the main course on wine pairing.

Do You Want Some Cheese with that Wine?

Go to any wine shop or wine lounge and you will inevitably encounter cheese selections alongside bottles or wine lists. Cheese and wine have gone together for thousands of years. There are many theories as to why this pair is seen as the perfect combination. Some make sense, some appear farfetched. One theory is that the fat and protein in cheese bond well with the components of wine and balance out the effects of alcohol. Others note that the saltiness of cheese naturally enhances the combination of alcohol and sugar in wine. Another more abstract idea is that both wine and cheese are the products of yeast fermentation, which creates a distinct taste reflecting where they are produced, like a geo-cultural marker. Maybe it's just a traditional thing like when people claim "they say…" without really knowing who "they" are or why "they" say something is so. Who knows for sure?

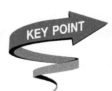

KEY POINT

Wine and cheese pair well for various reasons, most notably because of the balance between sweet and salty components.

Whatever the reason may really be, wine does get served with cheese regularly. A general guideline for choosing a wine and cheese combination is that the more rich and smelly the cheese, the sweeter the wine should be. That sounds easy enough, but what if you aren't a cheese expert? Buying cheeses can be as daunting, if not more so, than picking a wine. Cheese can be made from just about any type of milk from cow to reindeer (watch out Rudolph!) to yak. Each type of milk produces a different taste. Then there's the way it is all processed. Attempting to pair all wines and cheeses would be a job for a mathematician with roughly 10,000 varietals, countless blends, and a thousand or so chesses; it's mind blowing to try to understand all of the possible combinations.

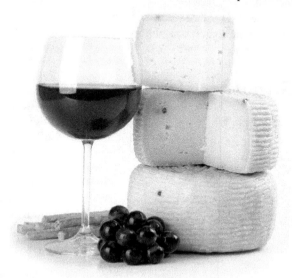

Let's stick to the basics. First, some general guidelines that will make things easier:

▶ For wines with higher tannin levels (bold reds), hard cheeses are appropriate.

▶ Creamy cheeses do best with wine that is more acidic (whites).

▶ Younger cheeses go well with fruity and crisp wines.

▶ Rich and heavy cheeses go well with lighter reds (Pinot Noir) and fuller Chardonnays.

▶ For cheeses with white or red rinds, a full white wine or soft reds work best.

▶ Strong, pungent, and veined cheeses (like Blue cheese) pair nicely with sweet and dessert wines.

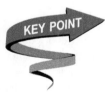

KEY POINT

To pair a cheese with a wine, use the acidity and fat content of the cheese as a guide. Light and creamy cheeses tend to go best with white wines. Hard cheeses pair better with red wines.

Cheese Pairings by Varietal

To take some of the guesswork out of your wine and cheese selections, this easy-to-follow guide will give you pairing combinations based on different wine varietals. The cheeses listed can be either easy to find in a typical grocery store or may take some extra hunting or a trip to a gourmet store for specialized suggestions.

Pinot Grigio/Pinot Gris

Pinot Grigio and Pinot Gris can range in taste from citrusy with lime and lemon notes to floral and honey with a bit of nectarine. The acidity typically present in these wines can provide a fuller feeling on the tongue that allows for a broader range of cheese pairings than with most white wines. For standard fare, Pinot Grigio pairs well with mild cheddar cheese. At the higher end of the orange-red cheese spectrum is a Red Leicester cheese, a cow's milk cheese similar to cheddar but with a higher moisture content, that does well with a Pinot Gris. Jarlsburg Light cheese (light because it is without a rind) has a sweet and nutty taste that goes well with the lighter varietal Pinot Grigio. Other white cheeses to consider with a Pinot Grigio are Appenzeller (nutty and fruity) and Apple Wood Smoked Gouda. Camembert, Chevre (tangy), Emmentaller, and Blue cheese (versions from cow's milk) work with both Pinot Grigio and Pinot Gris, but I personally prefer Pinot Gris with these cheeses.

Chardonnay

Chardonnay flavors range from young lemon and apple to ripened pineapple and mango. Wines aged in oak will also have buttery characteristics. With that in mind, oaked Chardonnay pairs well with creamier white cheeses. Pungent Brie varieties pair well with Chardonnay wines that are more ripe and tropical fruit forward. Asiago cheese works well across the Chardonnay spectrum as does Camembert. A pleasant taste surprise is an herb and garlic Chevre to balance a younger, non-oaked Chardonnay. Various types of Blue cheeses can work well, especially with wines that skew to the ripe fruit side. Gouda and Gruyere with sweet and nutty notes also compliment a variety of Chardonnay styles.

Gewürztraminer

The unique flavor profile of Gewürztraminer makes it the go-to pairing for some equally challenging cheeses. The wine's bouquet ranges from spicy grapefruit to lychee fruit. At its ripest end, the wine will have apricot and pineapple notes. Because of the range in fruit and spice, the Gewürztraminer can stand up to both orange and white cheddar cheeses. For those who like Swiss cheese, this wine pairs well with Jarlsburg and Jarlsburg Light cheeses. Swiss can be hard to pair with wine but this makes the best combination when you find it. Gouda, especially pungent Gouda made from goat's milk, is also a solid choice to go with Gewürztraminer selections.

Riesling

Pairing a Riesling with a cheese is tied directly to the nature of the wine itself. Rieslings can also run from citrusy in European bottles to nectarine and honey, especially in late harvest wines. The sweeter versions of Riesling pair well with medium to sharp cheddar cheeses. Mild or white cheddars are better matched with drier Rieslings. Milder Swiss cheese works across the different styles of Riesling too, especially an Emmentaller cheese with its nutty characteristics and milder taste. Mild Bleu cheeses work with Rieslings that skew towards the sweeter side. If you are looking for a wine to pair with a Mexican cheese like Cotija, a Riesling of any type is a good fit. Other cheeses that match up well with Rieslings are: Chevre, Fontina, Parmigiano Reggiano, Camembert, and Gouda.

Author's Aside

Before we move to the red varietals, I'd like to point out that wine and cheese doesn't have to be all snobbery. One of my favorite pick-me-ups or weeknight treats is to make a grilled cheese to go with my wine. It's a great comfort food and drink for that way too long week. A nice Asiago, Appenzeller, and Emmentaller grilled cheese with a cool Chardonnay or Pinot Grigio is a wonderful attitude adjustment. A classic cheddar cheese on sourdough bread with a Zinfandel is fabulous too. Who says you can't enjoy the simple things in life?

Pinot Noir

Moving to red wine varietals, Pinot Noir is the lightest of the reds with earthy and cranberry notes present in the Old World style of Pinot Noir. New World Pinots tend to be fruit forward with notes of cherry and raspberry. This is important to remember when pairing the wine with cheeses. For the earthier, European Pinot Noir, a Gruyere de Comté (or Comté as the shortened version) originates from near Burgundy, making it a geographical as well as a flavor match. Comté pairs well with this style of Pinot Noir, as well as being a very versatile cheese in its own right. Goat cheeses, such as Chevre, work well in addition to cheeses made from a combination of goat's and cow's milk. Other cheeses that pair favorably to Pinot Noir are: both white and smoked cheddar, Brie, and Gouda (the full range, and even the spicy versions that include chili peppers).

Author's Aside

On a winetasting trip to Napa a few years ago, I did a food pairing tasting at V. Sattui which matched a Pinot Noir with Sottocenere cheese. I have since forgotten all the other pairings because this morsel was absolutely delicious. Sottocenere is an Italian cheese flavored with flecks of truffle. It is to die for in combination with a Pinot Noir. The cheese matches nicely with earthy Pinot Noir from Burgundy, but I have to say it was phenomenal with a little fruiter California Pinot. The combination of cheese and truffle brought out the mushroom and earth in the wine for a balance that was otherwise easy to miss. The cheese is pricey because of the truffles, but it is definitely worth it in "Wow" factor.

Merlot

Merlots are at the midpoint of the red wine scale. They can be higher tannins, with an earthy and tobacco taste, or they can go in the opposite direction with lower tannin levels and more fruitiness. Because of this range, saltier cheeses tend to work best with Merlot. Mild orange and richer white cheddar work well with a Merlot wine that is fruit forward. Fontina is a good match with cooler, Old World Merlots because of its herb and fruity notes. Creamy Havarti works with both styles of Merlot, as does Gorgonzola. Additional selections include: Blue cheeses, Brie (particularly when baked with Portobello mushrooms inside), smoked Mozzarella, and smoked Provolone. For the extra adventurous, try Ricotta Salata. It is a Ricotta cheese that is dried to concentrate the saltiness of the sheep's milk it contains.

Zinfandel

Zinfandels tend to be very fruit forward, even jammy, and a bit peppery. As a result, bigger and bolder cheeses are often best with a glass of Zinfandel. Tangy cheddar cheeses work well with Zinfandel as does Aged Gouda. A stronger Gorgonzola works better to balance the wine than a milder cheese does. Manchego has a strong nutty flavor that packs a flavor punch with the fruit in the wine. Roquefort and Feta complete the Zinfandel pairings that work best across all styles of the wine.

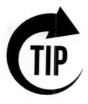 Because of the sweetness of White Zinfandel, spicy cheeses are wonderful pairs. Think Pepper Jack and related flavorful cheeses like cheddar with elements of peppers, herbs, and garlic.

Cabernet Sauvignon

Cabernets are known for cherry, currant, blackberry, black pepper, and even vanilla notes in the aroma and in the taste. While it can hold up when paired with a mild cheddar, the best cheese combinations are either sweet and nutty or bold. On the milder side, Asiago, Gruyere, and Fontina pair well with a more European-styled Cabernet Sauvignon. For fruitier New World Cabernets, Stilton and Bleu cheeses do best, but goat cheeses are also worth exploring as possible combinations, too.

Syrah

Because Syrah is an in-your-face type of wine, many think it pairs best with the strongest of cheeses, but that is not the case. To balance out the taste of a bold Syrah, the best cheeses to pair with it tend to be white with buttery or smoked flavors. Camembert is a better choice than Brie in the case of a Syrah because it is slightly richer, which holds up better against the wine. Provolone and Gouda are solid selections to pair with a Syrah. Even a Smoked Gouda or Smoked Mozzarella provides a pairing that enhances both the cheese and wine when put together.

TIP Add some fruit (berries and melons) or meats and olives to complete a little sampler platter with your wine. Cantaloupe and honeydew melons with Prosciutto or Serrano Ham go well with white wines and sparkling wines. Salami and other cured meats make a nice compliment to red wines. Bolder and fruiter reds are better with peppery meats. Also, olives are an alternative for pairings. Kalamata olives match nicely with Pinot Noir. Add a little Feta for a Mediterranean kick. California green olives make a good compliment to Chardonnay as well. Have some fun and experiment on your own.

Sparkling Wine

Because sparkling wines are effervescent and can range in sweetness levels, cheeses such as a creamy Gorgonzola, Camembert, and Brie work best. In the case of sweeter sparkling wines, a Parmigiano-Reggiano is a nice compliment. Sparkling wines can be one of the most versatile in pairing with cheeses, so it doesn't hurt to experiment with your personal preferences. Even an unlikely pairing with Marinated Feta can prove to be rewarding.

Ports and Dessert Wines

Because these wines are high in sugar and alcohol, cheeses need to be equally bold to balance out the tasting experience. For Ports, Bleu cheeses (including Stilton) work well, as do very sharp cheddars. For tawny Ports, the added element of brandy impacts the way it is paired with wine. A winning selection for a tawny Port is Pecorino Romano, aged if available is best. The sharp and tangy nature of the cheese counters the added alcohol in a tawny Port. A Madeira dessert wine goes nicely with a Gruyere because of complimentary nutty notes. For a dessert or Late Harvest Riesling, creamy Camembert and Muenster pair well, as do Swiss-style cheeses. A dessert-style Gewürztraminer opens up with Appenzeller because of the sharp fruity and slightly spicy nature of the cheese. A Muenster cheese also works well with a sweet Gewürztraminer.

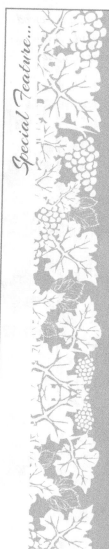

Special Feature...

Fromage Faux Pas

To look like you know what you're doing when serving cheeses, there is one golden rule: Do not serve chilly cheese. No, I'm not talking hot dogs here. Cheese should be served at room temperature. The full flavor of cheese develops at a warmer temperature. Guidelines vary from 30 minutes to an hour. For cheese wheels and larger blocks, a longer time is appropriate. Sliced cheese and smaller samples are fine with a half an hour to come up to temperature.

Also, cheese blocks and wheels should not be cut until they are ready to serve. If you have sliced cheese, the best thing to do is leave it in the wrapping until it is time to eat it so that it doesn't dry out. Purists will say you need a different knife for each type of cheese, but unless you slice a pungent one and then go to a mild one, this is not a hard and fast rule. A simple napkin wipe to clear the knife will do between slices.

The other question is: rind or no rind? Waxed rinds should never be eaten. Natural rinds are safe to eat, though many people do not like the texture or concentrated taste. When serving a cheese with a rind, do not remove the rind for service. If you are eating a cheese that has a rind that you do not want to eat, the polite thing to do is take rind with you. Don't leave it at the table for others to deal with. Just put it on your plate or discretely walk it to the nearest trash can for deposit.

Dish & Dinners

The most common task that wine drinkers face (aside from opening and consuming wine) is pairing meals, especially dinners, with wine. The general rule is white wine with white meats, salads, and seafood, and red wines with red meat. Of course, every rebel knows that rules are meant to be broken, so as the discussion of pairing varietals with dishes develops don't be surprised to see a few rebellious combinations included in the mix.

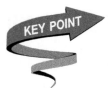

As a general rule, white wines go best with seafood, chicken, creamy pasta sauces, and salads. Red wines pair best with more flavorful pasta sauces, red meats, pork, and chocolates.

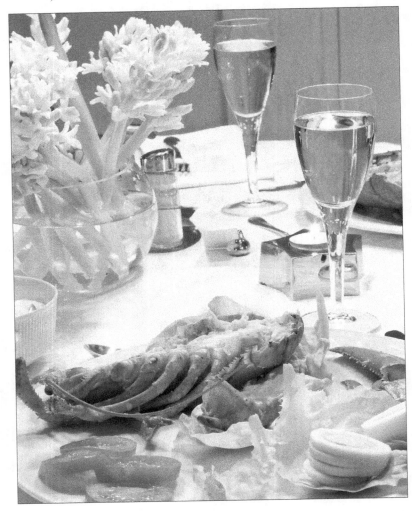

Sparkling Wine

While pairing sparkling wines with strawberries, oysters, and caviar is the most common way of serving food with sparkling wine, pairings do not have to be limited to appetizers or dessert trays. Buttery lobster dishes and lobster bisque match well with acidic sparkling wines. Egg dishes like omelets, scrambles, and quiches are always a solid choice for pairing with sparkling wines. (Is it any surprise with the popularity of Champagne brunches?) Butternut squash ravioli with a butter and sage sauce is an Italian themed alternative to a sparkling wine pairing. Spring rolls work well with bubbly too.

How about some "everyman/everywoman" fare for a bottle of sparkling wine? French fries are an unlikely combination for bubbly. Believe me, it works. A hint, eat fries with mayonnaise or ranch dressing instead of ketchup. A BBQ chicken sandwich with a tangy and spicy sauce balances lighter style sparkling wines. Even mac and cheese can pair with bubbly if it uses medium, creamy cheeses like Gouda, white American, and Parmesan. Ham, truffles, or lobster can be added to mac and cheese to round out the dish.

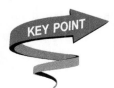

KEY POINT *Sparkling wine pairings are not limited to appetizer and dessert trays.*

Pinot Gris/Pinot Grigio

The overall theme for Pinot Gris and Pinot Grigio is veggies, white meats, and seafood. Lighter salads featuring vegetables like cucumber, squash, celery, onion, kale, green apple, honeydew melon, cauliflower, and broccoli do well with Pinot Grigio. Creamy salad dressings work better with Pinot Grigio rather than Pinot Gris because of a characteristically higher alcohol content and a

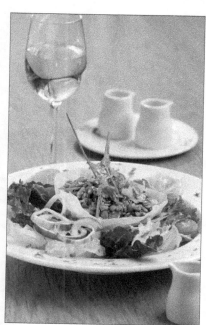

fuller body. Meat dishes featuring chicken, turkey and spiced duck or pork pair beautifully with both wines. Seafood such as tilapia, bass, sole, trout, cod, halibut, and snapper in addition to calamari, scallops, mussels, oysters, and clams are common dishes served with Pinot Grigio or Pinot Gris. The wine also makes a perfect go-to choice for more raw seafood options such as ceviche and sushi.

Because the characteristics of Pinot Gris favor spices like mint, tarragon, parsley, coriander, fennel, turmeric, and saffron, it matches well with Indian, Moroccan, and Greek food. Lighter Italian fare such as pasta primavera and pesto dishes go well with Pinot Gris, while white and cream sauces such as Alfredo and Carbonara are better suited to Pinot Grigio to lighten the palate.

More specific pairings of food with Pinot Grigio and Pinot Gris that bring out both the food and wine include Greek salads and tabouli because of the concentration of parsley and other herbs. A ratatouille rich in tarragon, onions, and squash can be a French-influenced dish to go with Pinot Gris. Turkey and chicken sausages work well with Pinot Grigio because of both the meat and the typical use of fennel and coriander in sausage spices and those that have apple in them are even a better match with the wine. If you prefer wine to beer with your fish and chips, Pinot Grigio is the option to consider.

Ham, truffles, or lobster can be added to mac and cheese to round out the dish.

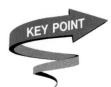

KEY POINT

Pinot Grigio and Pinot Gris are the best matches for salads, vegetables, and seafood.

Chardonnay

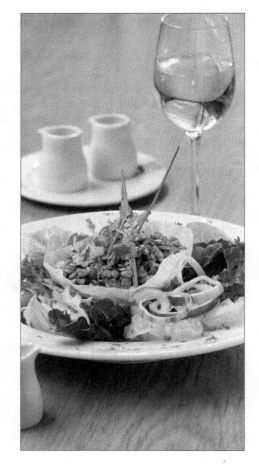

Chardonnay is considered the universal white wine as well as the go-to choice for white meat chicken and turkey, pork loin, and seafood. Fish that is flaky and oily is suited to this white wine, but surprisingly so are other seafood options such as salmon, lobster, crab, shrimp, scallops, and clams. In the case of oysters, an un-oaked version of Chardonnay works best. The optimal vegetable pairings are more limited with Chardonnay than with Pinot Grigio. Mushrooms such as truffles, button, and chanterelles are the best combinations. Zucchini, summer squash, peas, and asparagus also do well with Chardonnay, as do almonds. Dishes with thyme and other poultry seasonings in addition to tarragon, marjoram, shallots, and lemon zest are suited to Chardonnay pairings. It stands to reason that lemon chicken-based meals do well with a Chardonnay to add some palate cleaning acid to the tasting experience. However, a less likely pairing of Chardonnay with fried chicken is a good comfort food combination. Butter-based seafood entrees pair nicely with Chardonnay, though an un-oaked wine may be more appropriate to balance flavors than a wine that has the buttery influences of oak.

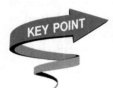

Chardonnay pairs well with white meats and flaky and oil seafood.

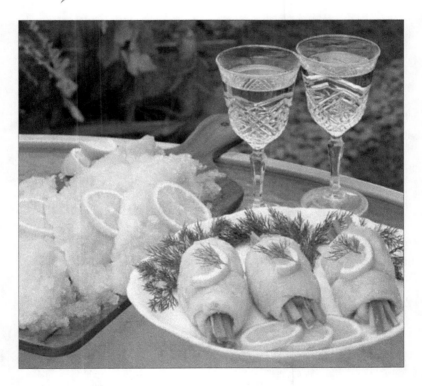

Gewürztraminer

Gewürztraminer is the match to many dishes that would otherwise be viewed as hard to pair with wine because the wine stands up well to spices. Ingredients such as cayenne pepper, coriander, and cumin, which are common in south of the border dishes, combine well with the wine. Curry in Indian food pops with a flavor surprise when paired with a Gewürztraminer. Asian foods with ginger, allspice, Sichuan pepper, shallots, soy sauce, sesame, and almond also benefit from the wine. Meats that pair with Gewürztraminer range from duck and chicken (especially the dark meat) to pork and bacon, and shellfish such as crab and shrimp. Given the overall tendencies for successful pairings with Gewürztraminer, it is common to see the wine served with Mexican, Indian, and Asian entrees.

Even with vegetables, Gewürztraminer pairs with otherwise challenging food items such as artichokes. Red onion, bell pepper, eggplant, squash, carrots, and parsnips also combine well with the wine. Roasting a selection of these vegetables brings out more of their sugars, further enhancing the taste of a Gewürztraminer. Also, the sweetness of coconut, be it the flesh or the milk, makes a pleasing match with the wine for both dinner and dessert dishes.

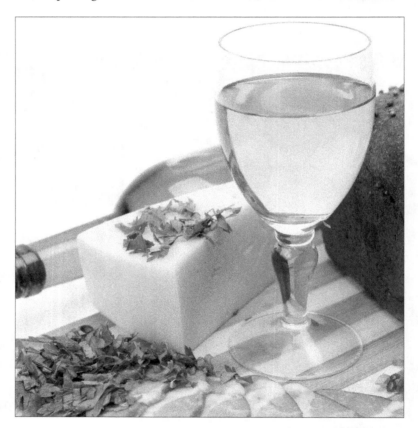

Riesling

Riesling and Gewürztraminer share many pairing characteristics for meat, vegetables, spices, and specific ethnic dishes. Rieslings do offer some additional options though. For Thai food and Asian dishes that feature teriyaki sauce or rice vinegar, Riesling is the better wine selection of the two. Ham that is seasoned with clove and pork dishes served with apples are also better suited to this wine. Yellowtail and salmon sushi pop with Rieslings, as does red clam chowder.

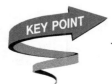

Gewürztraminer and Riesling have similar food pairing characteristics and are good for spicy ethnic dishes.

Author's Aside

Believe it or not, Riesling makes a perfect tailgating wine. The unlikely pairing of Riesling and Bratwurst provides a tasty alternative to beer. Also, Riesling pairs nicely with spicy buffalo wings and guacamole, of all things. For the adventurous tailgater or couch quarterback, Riesling works well in and with fondue (especially cheddar based). I know firsthand. I've done it at tailgates at the Rose Bowl. Bring on the football!

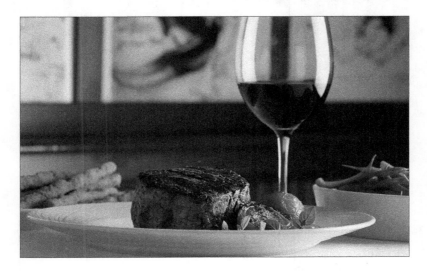

Pinot Noir

Pinot Noir is truly the go-to red wine for dishes that are not especially spicy. It pairs with everything from a burger that has mustard and relish to white pizzas and pizza with olives, onions, mushrooms and ham, to Gnocchi, corned beef, or rabbit. The flavor range in Pinot Noir, from earthy European selections to fruity wines from the United States, allows the wine to be highly versatile with food matches. Pinot Noir wines work well with pork, chicken, beef (roasted or braised), and duck. Mushrooms, broccoli, asparagus, peas, and olives pair with both New and Old World-style wines, as do breads and savory pastry dishes. Pinot Noir breaks the white wine with seafood rule by creating a balanced pairing with lobster, salmon, and even fettuccine Alfredo. This wine is perfect

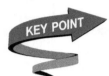

with Thanksgiving dishes like cornbread stuffing, scalloped potatoes, Brussel sprouts au gratin, and green bean casseroles. Herbs and spices that work well in dishes served with Pinot Noir include chives, rosemary, herbs de Provence, garlic, thyme, poultry seasonings, and pepper. Even peanut-based Thai dishes and peanut brittle work with Pinot Noir.

KEY POINT *Pinot Noir can be one of the most versatile red wines for food pairings.*

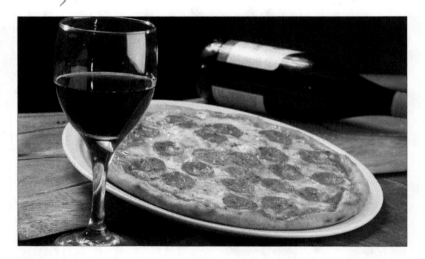

Merlot

Merlot is a wine that does not pair well with green leafy vegetables or the majority of seafood. Instead, Merlot is an ideal match for tomato-based dishes featuring chicken, pork chops, beef, and lamb. Minestrone and tomato soup also provide a flavorful combination. This wine is also the perfect match to heartier beef dishes, from meatballs to burgers and French dip sandwiches to steak. Mexican food dishes such as chicken enchiladas, quesadillas, and huevos rancheros pair with the wine due in part to onions and peppers that are often included in these dishes. Stuffed peppers and mushrooms with beef, lamb, and even tuna, as well as pizza topped with shrimp, onions, and peppers accentuate a Merlot. A shepherd's pie does well with the wine, especially when lamb is used. For a dessert option, pair a Merlot with a chocolate soufflé.

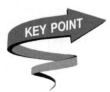

KEY POINT *Merlot wines generally do not pair well with leafy vegetables or seafood but match nicely with tomato-based dishes.*

TIP To neutralize sweetness in tomato sauces, add a half glass to full glass of Merlot or Zinfandel to the sauce while it is simmering. The alcohol will evaporate and leave the sauce with tannins and acidity that will balance out the sweetness in the sauce and add a dimension to the overall taste.

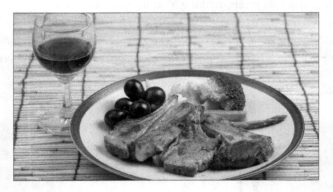

Zinfandel

Meat dishes that pair well with a Zinfandel run the spectrum from spiced up turkey and pork, to ham and bacon, to barbecued beef items, and lamb or veal. To match vegetables with a Zinfandel and maximize the fruitiness of the wine, roasting is the best option. Try roasting tomatoes, red peppers, and onion in dishes served with Zins. Roasted squash from summer squash and zucchini to butternut and spaghetti squash do well with the wine. Even fruits such as cranberries, spiced apples, apricots, and peaches can enhance a Zinfandel's taste.

The flexibility of Zinfandel as a wine is reflected in the spices and herbs that work with the wine. Powerful spices such as curry, turmeric, saffron, and cayenne pepper make Zinfandel the red wine choice for Indian food and similar dishes. Ginger, clove, nutmeg, cinnamon, vanilla, and cocoa allow for Zinfandel to match with dessert dishes while the trio of black pepper, garlic, and rosemary make it friendly for red meat fare.

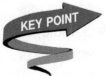

Zinfandel pairs with meats from turkey to BBQ and cured meats and roasted veggies.

Cabernet Sauvignon

Cabernet Sauvignon is an excellent wine for all things beef, whether it is a stew, pot roast, burger, or steak. Fleshy fish like tuna, swordfish, and shark stand up to the chewiness of a Cabernet as well. Venison, pheasant, buffalo, ostrich, and lamb are balanced with a Cabernet in either the Old World or New World traditions. On the other hand, a peppery herb duck dish featuring mushrooms works best with Cab wines from the United States. Vegetables generally do not pair well with the high tannins in a Cabernet, with the exception of peppery and spicy arugula and radicchio for salads as well as eggplant. There is a bonus with Cab pairings. It is the wine for anything, and I do mean anything, that has chocolate in it.

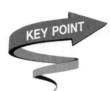

KEY POINT *Cabernet Sauvignon is a compliment to beef and gamier meat dishes, as well as all types of chocolate.*

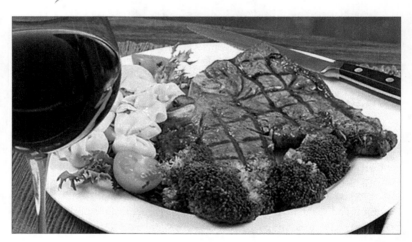

TIP Given that Cabernet Sauvignon is typically paired with beef and gamier meats, it may be a surprise to learn of a chicken dish that is ideal for the wine. Chicken mole, with the dark sauce, makes for an unexpected and successful match to a Cabernet. The traditional black mole, a sauce originating in Mexico, contains small amounts of chocolate which is one reason the dish works.

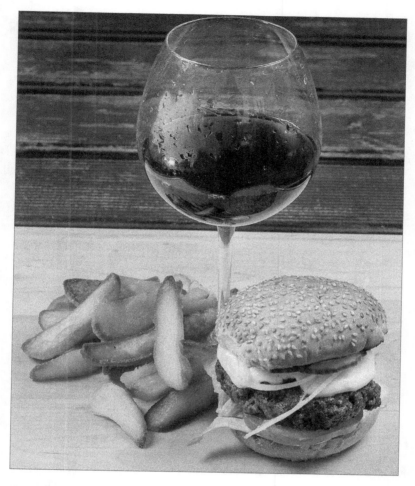

Syrah

Like Cabernet Sauvignon, Syrah's high tannin levels do not pair well with vegetables. The possible exceptions to that rule are tomatoes, flavorful mushrooms, and potatoes that balance the wine. For meat and potato lovers, that works out well because Syrah is the big bad BBQ wine that pairs best with grilled or roasted red meats. Seasonings such as garlic, onion, pepper, and rosemary do well with both red meats and the wine. In addition to red meats, highly seasoned pork and cured meats can be paired with Syrah successfully.

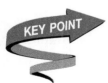

KEY POINT

Syrah is the "Big Bad BBQ" wine that overwhelms nearly all vegetables and lighter meat fare.

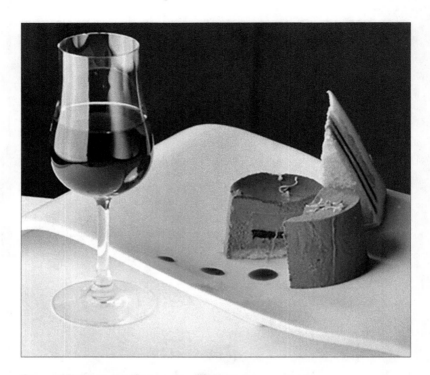

Port Wine & Dessert Wine

Port wines and dessert wines are typically served with desserts and other sweets rather than with entrees because food dishes are overpowered by the concentrated flavors in these selections. However, Port is a popular addition to many dishes when used as a reduction. To make a Port wine reduction, the wine is poured into a pan and heated slowly until the liquids thicken into a syrupy consistency. One way to incorporate Port into a meal is through a pork roast. Raisins soaked in Port overnight and allowed to plump up can be poured over roasting pork to provide sweetness to the roast (similar to using apples.)

Ports and dessert wines can be served with cheese, nuts, and dessert trays, but they can also be incorporated into the desserts themselves. Baked apples or pears can be basted in a Port with the addition of spices such as cinnamon and nutmeg. In warmer weather, ice wines and specialty flavored ports (like chocolate or raspberry) can be drizzled over ice cream or a pound cake topped with fruit as a final course.

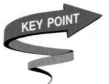

Port and dessert wines are not typically served with entrees but can be used as an ingredient in dishes.

THE TAKEAWAY

Wine and food has been a match made in heaven since the beginning of wine drinking time. While some wines seem to beg for particular wine partners, others benefit from a wider selection of pairing opportunities. Some food can be challenging to match with wine, but that is simply part of the fun for a wine lover. George Carlin once asked "What wine goes with Captain Crunch?" Sure, he was probably just being his sarcastic self, but to those who enjoy wine, it presents a fun challenge. You don't have to memorize everything in this section and what goes with what. Instead, use this like you would a cookbook.

Take your favorite foods and play. Some pairings will make you do a little dance while others may make you shudder. That's the fun of wine: it's a participation sport that includes an enjoyable learning process. **Here are the key points from the chapter:**

► Wine and cheese pair well because of the balance between sweet and salty components.

► To pair a cheese with a wine, use the acidity and fat content of the cheese as a guide. Light and creamy cheeses tend to go best with white wines. Hard cheeses pair better with red wines.

► As a general rule, white wines go best with seafood, chicken, creamy pasta sauces, and salads.

► As a general rule, red wines pair best with more flavorful pasta sauces, red meats, pork, and chocolates.

► There are exceptions to the general the white and red rules.

► Sparkling wine pairings are not limited to appetizer and dessert trays.

► Pinot Gris and Grigio are the best matches for salads, vegetables, and seafood.

► Chardonnay pairs well with white meats and flaky and oily seafood.

► Gewürztraminer and Riesling have similar food pairing characteristics and are good for spicy ethnic dishes.

► Pinot Noir is the most versatile red wine for food pairings.

► Merlot wines generally do not pair well with leafy vegetables or seafood but match nicely with tomato-based dishes.

► Zinfandel pairs with meats from turkey to BBQ and cured meats and roasted veggies.

► Cabernet Sauvignon is a compliment to beef and gamier meat dishes as well as all types of chocolate.

► Syrah is the "Big Bad BBQ" wine that overwhelms nearly all vegetables and lighter meat fare.

► Port and dessert wines are not typically served with entrees but can be used as an ingredient in dishes.

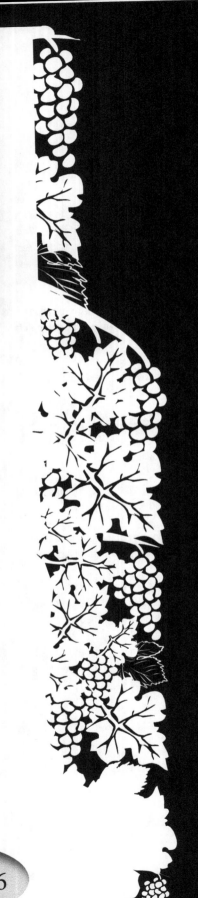

*"Always carry a corkscrew, and
the wine shall provide itself."*

—Basil Bunting

4

Tools of the Trade

Wine tools come in a variety of shapes, sizes, and functions. Some are required. Some are useful. Some are simply for fun or novelty. The reality of it all is that you need, at the very least, a way to open the bottle (for those bottles that have a cork) and something to drink the wine from. In truly desperate times, even those two necessities can be discarded—you just get a twist-off bottle and drink from the bottle itself. Yes, I said it. It's not just for winos on benders. Think of how many times a winning race car driver has gulped bubbly straight from the bottle in Victory Lane. Sometimes you've just gotta do what you gotta do.

All jesting aside, those who want to experience wine will need certain "accoutrements" to make the wine tasting and drinking experience the best it can be. Wine tools fall into four basic categories: openers, decanters, glasses, and storage items. After learning about options to open a bottle of wine, we will briefly touch on a range of decanting options. We'll cover the most perplexing aspect of wine for beginners, glasses, and answer the popular question: "Why is my wine served in a glass shaped like this?" The final part of this section will cover storage options for those who can delay instant gratification with their vino.

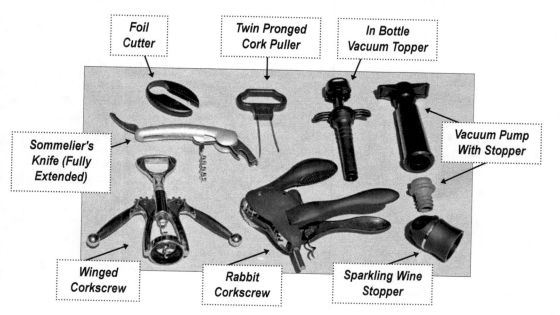

Foil Cutter

Twin Pronged Cork Puller

In Bottle Vacuum Topper

Sommelier's Knife (Fully Extended)

Vacuum Pump With Stopper

Winged Corkscrew

Rabbit Corkscrew

Sparkling Wine Stopper

Corkscrews and Openers

TIP Wing corkscrews are also known as butterfly corkscrews or, my personal favorite, angel corkscrews. Anyone looking for a glass of wine after a rough day can appreciate the angelic quality of this opener to help turn the day or evening around with a simple pop.

Corkscrews have evolved from the classic T-shape form with a wooden handle and metal corkscrew end to a variety of items that make it even easier to get wine from the bottle to the glass. The traditional corkscrews today are made of metal and/or plastic and come in two forms. One of the most common corkscrews is referred to as a wing corkscrew, which is a combination bottle opener and wine opener. It has a ring that sits around the mouth of the bottle with the screw end that twists down into the cork as arms at the side of the opener rise with each turn. When the curls of the corkscrew are completely in the cork, the arms can be pushed down to pull the cork out of the bottle. A final tug on the corkscrew often will be necessary to completely remove the cork from the bottle (with a rewarding "pop.")

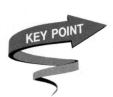

KEY POINT *The winged corkscrew is the most common corkscrew.*

The second most common type of corkscrew is the sommelier's knife, which is also known as the waiter's friend or a wine key. It folds up to look like a modified pocket knife but contains a small knife for remove foil from the top of wine bottles, a stepped arm to provide to provide leverage, and a corkscrew point. The sommelier's knife takes a little more skill to learn how to use than the winged corkscrew and can require a little more "oomph" for cork extraction. However, it allows for more of a show when opening a bottle in front of an audience.

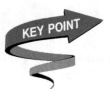

KEY POINT *The sommelier knife or wine key is the second most common corkscrew and requires a little more practice to use than a winged corkscrew.*

The twin prong cork puller, also known as the butler's friend, is a third corkscrew option. The selling point to this type of corkscrew is that the cork can be removed without damage to allow it to be re-inserted later. The two prongs are designed to slide between the glass in the bottle neck and the cork.

To reverse the process, the prongs can be used to put the cork back in the bottle. The cork is placed between the prongs and twisted back into the bottle. The prongs then slide out once the cork is replaced.

TIP Though convenient for travel, under current TSA regulations, a sommelier's knife is not allowed in carry-on luggage when flying. It will need to be stowed in checked luggage or sacrificed at the obligatory security checkpoint. I've lost several after forgetting about them in my purse, so consider this a helpful FYI.

Author's Aside

I have personally had limited success with the pronged cork puller. Part of that may be because I use it when trying to open older bottles with potentially damaged corks. The reality is that any damage to the cork from either a winged corkscrew or a sommelier knife does not preclude using the cork as a stopper. One problem that you may encounter when reusing the cork as a stopper is that the cork will expand once it leaves the bottle, making it difficult to reinsert. A simple solution is to turn the cork upside down, putting the dry end inside the bottle, when reinserting it as a stopper. Any expansion due to moisture will be most evident on the end that was in contact with the wine, so using the other end avoids that issue.

Other forms of corkscrews and openers have come on the market to fill a variety of needs. Some are designed to insert compressed gas into the bottle to force the cork out. Recently, the sale of such models has been halted due to safety concerns with bottles shearing and causing injury. Corkscrews that are modifications of the winged opener have become popular, with the more popular Rabbit openers. Rabbit-style openers have two arms that wrap around the neck of the wine bottle. A third arm comes down with the screw tip, goes into the cork, and is then pulled back up to remove the cork. For those with conditions such as arthritis or weaker hand/arm strength, these types of openers can be easier to use with the difference in leveraging.

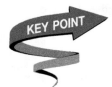

Specialized corkscrews and wine openers are available to assist those who otherwise have difficulty uncorking a bottle.

Decanters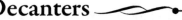

Now that you have conquered the biggest challenges of getting a bottle of wine and opening it, it is time to address the more refined points to enjoying wine. In many cases, there will be a need to **decant** the wine prior to pouring a glass, in order to allow it to **breathe** and open up. Though patience is required, decanters allow for a "time out" for the wine in order to open up and reach its fruity and tasty best. It sounds snobbish, and there are indeed ways to decant wine that take the process over the top and into elitism. However, decanting is just plain good sense, and can be done in budget-friendly ways.

Shop Talk...

17. **Decant** [DE-cant], verb. The process of taking wine from a bottle and placing it in a container to sit for a period of time before serving wine in a glass. The container used is referred to as a decanter. Older and unfiltered wines may have sediment that will need to settle to the bottom of a decanter before pouring to avoid a sludge coating in the glass. Younger wines can also benefit from sitting in a decanter to get increased exposure to oxygen prior to serving.

18. **Breathe**, verb. The process of letting a wine rest and come in contact with air in order to let the aroma and flavors open up for maximum taste. Think of letting your wine breathe as similar to how you feel when you climb from your car after a long road trip. After a long ride, you need to stretch and flex your muscles to move freely once again. The same is true for your wine. It needs to expand after being confined in the bottle before it will be at its best.

Decanter Options

At the most basic level, a decanter is a container that is larger than a wine bottle that allows more of the surface of the wine to come into contact with the air. They are fun wine accessories to have when serving at gatherings too. Decanters are typically designed with a wide base and a narrow neck. The narrow opening helps keep any sediment in the wine out of the glass. They come in a wide range of shapes and sizes. A carafe is a common style of decanter used in restaurants. While glass is the material of choice, high-end decanters can be made of crystal.

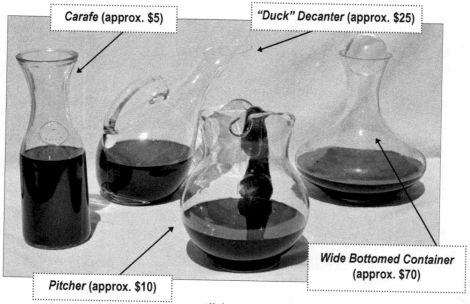

All decanters contain a full bottle of wine.

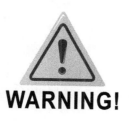

WARNING!

Leaded crystal decanters are not appropriate for long-term storage of wine. Studies have shown that the lead, which poisonous even at the 1% level, can leech into the wine, which also means it can get into your body. Short-term use of leaded crystal, as in glasses or decanters where the wine is consumed in a single event (like dinner) won't hurt you, but leaving it in there too long exposes you to the risk of lead ingestion.

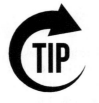

You don't have to go out and spend tens or hundreds of dollars on a decanter to decant your wine. I often forego my decanter and simply use a pitcher for informal, no-nonsense wine drinking. I have used both glass and plastic pitchers with the same success as my traditional decanter, though I prefer glass.

Wine Glasses

Glassware is usually more interesting and important to those beginning with wine. Have you ever wondered why a red wine is served in a glass that is different from a white wine glass? How about the shape of Champagne glasses? Now, hopefully, you will understand that there is indeed some sort of method to the wine glass madness.

Elements of a Wine Glass

Wine glasses have three elements: the base, the stem, and the bowl.

The **base** is the area that rests on a table. It supports the glass and allows it to remain upright. The stem is the long thin "neck" of the glass that does not hold wine. While it may be pretty and distinctive among glassware, it does have a purpose.

The **stem** allows the drinker to hold the glass without transferring body heat to the wine. It also allows the glass to be held without creating smudges on the bowl that can distract from the look of the wine in the glass. Of course, there's an exception to every rule, and the newer stemless glasses that are shaped as a tumbler do not have a stem; the base of these glasses is also part of the bowl itself.

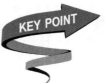

Decanting wine is the process of pouring a bottle of wine into a large container before serving in a wine glass. That allows the wine to breathe and lets sediment settle before pouring.

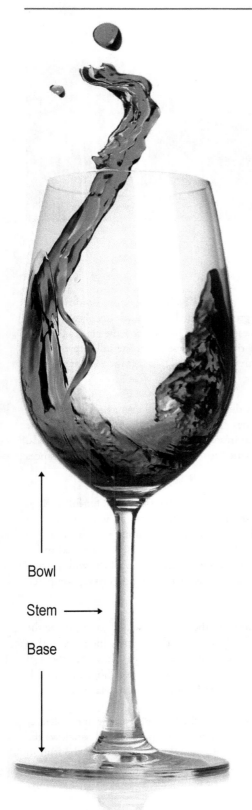

Bowl

Stem →

Base

The **bowl**, the area that actually holds the wine, is the most distinctive part of a wine glass. It is also where the greatest level of variation comes from in glassware. Glasses will have a narrower opening at the top than the bottom. Some will be more so than others. The same holds true for the width and depth of the bottom of the bowl.

The differences in design serve an important purpose in fully enjoying the wine in each type of glass. The shapes are used to capture and distribute a wine's aroma for the nose and mouth.

Glassware
Shapes and Sizes

There are more than two dozen wine glass shapes that are designed for different purposes. On top of that, countless other shapes are produced simply for novelty.

The easiest way to understand wine glass shapes is to note four general categories:

red, white, sparkling, and dessert.

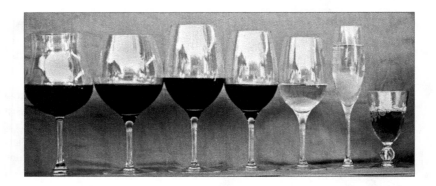

Red Wine Glasses

Glasses used for red wines such as Pinot Noir, Burgundy, Bordeaux, and Zinfandel are larger and are, as a group, referred to as Bordeaux glasses by tradition. The opening of these glasses are larger than white wine glasses to allow the drinker to dip a nose into the rim of the glass to get the full impact of the wine's aroma. These taller glasses are also designed to target the wine at the back of the mouth for maximum flavor.

A Pinot Noir glass (pictured on the left) is designed to maximize the enjoyment of the lightest of the red wines. The deep and wider bowl help the wine open up to its full aroma and flavor in some of the most delicate of all the reds. The ridge near the lip helps the wine hit the tongue in an area that enhances the experience of fruit in each sip.

A Burgundy glass (pictured second from the left) is designed for fuller Pinot Noir wines. It has the same depth and width to allow the wine to open in regard to flavor and aroma, but it does not have the additional ridge near the lip. Without the ridge, wine sipped from a Burgundy glass is allowed to hit the tongue farther back to allow drinkers experience more of the wine's structure through the more pronounced tannins that Burgundies have, compared to other Pinot Noir wines.

A Bordeaux glass (pictured third from the left) is designed to maximize the aromas and flavors in Cabernet Sauvignon. It is the largest wine glass, with a more elongated bowl. The larger bowl and wider mouth allow the aroma of these big-bodied red wines to develop and to expand throughout the glass. It also lets the wine hit the tongue farther back for a fuller taste experience.

A Zinfandel glass (pictured fourth from the left) is a smaller, more slender version of a Bordeaux glass. The more pointed shape of the glass allows the wine to hit the tongue in the mid-palate area to highlight more of the fruit in the wine. The bowl enables the aroma to expand and concentrate in the glass. A Zinfandel glass can also be used as a white wine glass that has a larger volume.

White Wine Glasses

White wine glasses (pictured third from the right) are generally smaller than red wine glasses because white wines are better when sipped at cooler temperatures. The size helps with smaller pours that be consumed before the wine warms. White wine glasses have a rounded bowl with a more upright shape than a Zinfandel glass. The lip of the glass does not curve inward because of the nature of aromas in white wines—they are more forward from the time the wine is poured, meaning the aromas are present almost immediately. The straighter lip also causes the wine to hit the middle of the palate, to emphasize the acid while still featuring the wine's fruit.

Sparkling Wine Glasses

Sparkling wine glasses (pictured second from the right), also known as flutes, are among the narrowest wine glasses, though the curve of the flute can vary. Some flutes are nearly vertical while others have a slightly tulip-like shape. Aroma is not as critical when drinking sparkling wines, so the narrow opening is designed to retain carbonation while directing flavor to the sides and tip of the tongue when sipped.

Author's Aside

I've been asked about what could be considered "must have" glasses. For those on a budget or truly just starting out with wine, I suggest 4-6 red wine glasses (Zinfandel glasses are the most universal). In reality, for most everyday situations, a red wine glass will cover just about every type of wine service. Heck, I've even used them for sparkling wines (and mimosas). If you are going to drink sparkling wine on a regular basis, I would suggest breaking down and investing in 2-6 sparkling wine flutes, depending on the number of people you typically pop the cork with. There's just something to having sparkling wine from the proper glass during social functions, and flutes can be found at reasonable prices for any budget.

Dessert Wine Glasses

Glasses designed for dessert wines (pictured on the right) will be smaller versions of a wine glass and can take a variety of shapes. Because dessert wines have high levels of sweetness, glasses are designed to allow wine to hit the back of the mouth so that the sweetness does not overwhelm the tasting process. Also, dessert wines tend to have higher levels of alcohol, so the smaller glass provides the proper serving size.

Other Wine Glasses

Of course, there is a plethora of other shapes and sizes for wine glasses within each of the four categories. For example, sparkling wine can be served in coupe or vintage (a wide and shallow bowl) as opposed to a flute or tulip-shaped glass. Ports can be served in a traditional Port glass or in some cases a small brandy snifter.

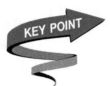 *Wine glasses come in a variety of shapes and sizes to maximize the tasting experience of a particular type or style of wine.*

Crystal Not-So-Clear

Spend any time in the wine world and you will find that people have particular views about the benefits of using crystal versus traditional glassware for wine tasting. Some wine lovers believe that wine tastes better in crystal as opposed to in glass. The science behind that view is somewhat debatable. Currently, the accepted belief is that crystal has a rougher surface structure than regular glass. The speculation is that the roughness causes the wine's aroma to be released more fully when it travels over crystal. Also, part of the wine tasting experience is a visual one. Thinner crystal glasses allow the clarity and color of a wine to be experienced more fully compared to a thicker glass. A final argument for the use of crystal rather than glass is that crystal creates a finer stream of wine while sipping than that of traditional glass. The benefit there is said to be that it creates a better a mixture between air, wine, and taste buds.

One of the greatest concerns regarding the use of leaded crystal is the potential of lead leeching into wine. Riedel, a leading manufacturer of crystal glassware, addressed the issue as follows:

"Today the word 'lead' has a negative connotation. However the 'lead' oxide in glass is totally integrated into the molecular structure, which enables us to continue to use it. Regarding lead leeching, worldwide legal standards are met and also surpassed. This legal and official authorization, which allows the production of drinking vessels executed in lead crystal, proves that consumers may use lead crystal on a daily basis and do not need to be concerned about any risk to health."[1]

I think it's a personal call based on your preferences, concerns, and budget. I have a few crystal pieces, but I've found that the wine glasses that I

[1] http://www.riedel.com/all-about-riedel/what-is-lead-crystal/ "What is Lead Crystal?" Riedel, 2014

got for $3 apiece work just as well as the crystal pieces that cost four times as much. I have to admit, it is nice to have a little splurge glassware for major celebrations, but it's up to you.

Wine Storage

While the overall focus of this book is on the experience of drinking wine, storage is both a short-term and long-term concern for those who buy wine. You don't need to store wine for decades in order to find some knowledge in the dos and don'ts of wine storage useful. For our purposes, storage includes everything from getting the wine home to handling wine leftovers to longer-term storage. Wine storage begins at the moment you purchase your bottle.

Like pets and children, wine should never be left in a hot car. Heat and sunlight are detrimental to wine and cause changes in the appearance and the taste of wine. Purchases should be taken home and stored in a cool dark place. If you purchase wine that can't be taken home immediately, you can extend the transit time and minimize damage to your wine by keeping an ice chest in your vehicle. You don't have to put ice in it. The ice chest can provide a temperature buffer and placing any cool or frozen items in with your wine will provide additional cooling. If you don't have an ice chest, covering wine bottles to avoid both sunlight and to provide some degree of insulation can help keep your wine "happy" for a longer period of time. Once you have taken your wine home, it should be placed in a cool place out of direct sunlight. If wine is to be consumed immediately, it can be placed in a refrigerator to chill as soon as you get home.

KEY POINT *Never "cook" your wine by leaving it in a hot car or other hot environment.*

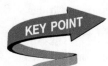

A common question for those new to wine is: how do I store an open bottle? An open bottle can be stored in the refrigerator for several days. A stopper should be inserted into the bottle to avoid more oxygenation that will cause the wine to deteriorate. Stoppers can be as simple as reusing the original cork. Other types of stoppers that help preserve wine for longer periods use a vacuum pump which pulls out the air from the bottle and leaves a rubber stopper in place. There is also a selection of wine preservers that can be shot or sprayed into a bottle to keep the wine fresher for longer. However, the wine may be damaged by the addition of preservatives.

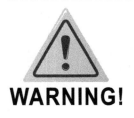

WARNING!

Never remove the metal cage on a sparkling wine bottle and let it sit without removing the cork. The gases in sparkling wine cause pressure to build and eject the cork on its own. This can cause injury or damage. The same is true for "re-corking" sparkling wines with anything other than stoppers specifically designed for sparkling wine bottles.

Special Feature...

Stick A Fork In It?

Well, a silver spoon would be more a more appropriate instrument in this case. As noted in the previous warning, open bottles of sparkling wine require a different approach to short-term storage. Ideally, you should aim to finish a bottle of sparkling wine within 1-2 hours after it is opened. That allows you to get the best tasting and most effervescent experience, but that is not always feasible. A popular piece of French folklore states that putting a silver spoon, handle down, into an open bottle of sparkling wine will keep it fresh and bubbly for days. A group of researchers at Stanford University put the wives' tale to the test by using both silver and stainless steel spoons. After 26 hours in a fridge, the best of the partial bottles of sparkling wines were those that were left completely open. The second best were the ones with a spoon inserted into the bottle. It didn't matter if the spoon was made silver or stainless steel. Finally, "recorking" was found to be the worst way to keep the bubbly…bubbly. The researchers were not able to achieve the statistical significance that academics strive for to say the testing was scientifically valid, but the results were later confirmed by the Centre Interprofesionel des Vins de Champagne in France. So much for folklore!

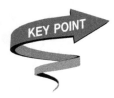

KEY POINT

Wine glasses come in a variety of shapes and sizes to maximize the tasting experience of a particular type or style of wine.

Long-Term Storage

Let's say that you receive bottles of wine as gifts or find a killer deal on your favorite vino and decide to stock up on it. The storage task shifts from preparing for drinking to finding a wine-friendly space within your abode. There is definitely a right way to store wine and plenty of wrong ways to do so. We've all been there. You walk into someone's kitchen (of course, not your own) and look above the refrigerator to find a collection of wine bottles. Then you look to the other side of the kitchen and see a wine rack, filled with bottles hanging from the cabinet, above the stove. If you were polite, you hid the grimace and maybe offered to move the bottles. If you didn't grimace, now you'll know why you should have.

Those who begin to keep wine for longer than it takes to finish the next meal will learn quickly that wine should be stored at a specific temperature. In fact, the perfect temperature for cellaring or storing wine is about 55 degrees. Notice the word "perfect." In fact, extensive research has been done regarding the impact of temperatures ranging from 55 to 91 degrees. The findings suggested that one month of wine aging/storage at 91 degrees equals roughly 4 months to 18 years of aging at 55 degrees. Consider a typical average room temperature of 73 degrees. Storing your wine at room temperature versus the ideal temperature of 55 degrees makes wine age anywhere from 2 to 8 times faster. That means, storing your wine for 3 years at room temperature will age your wine anywhere from 6 to 24 years faster. Yes, if you are storing a high-end wine for the long haul, then a temperature in the 50s is important. In most cases, however, keeping it in a cool and dark environment will be fine for those who consume their wine bottles on a regular basis.

Humidity levels are also noted in proper wine storage procedures. Those who store wines for longer periods of time (a decade or more) do need to be concerned with keeping the cork from drying out over the long haul. In these cases, keeping a humidity level at 70% is important. Generally speaking, storing a bottle in environments that have between 50% and 80% humidity will otherwise be fine. Since I live in an area that regularly sees low humidity levels, I simply add a pan of water to the bottom of my wine closet, which evaporates naturally. When the humidity is in the single digits, I call in the big guns and add a humidifier, but that is only because I do have several bottles that have rested in my collection for a decade or more. If you regularly drink your wine and keep the bottles rotated by the date purchased, your wine will be fine without added moisture measures.

You don't need a fancy wine cellar to keep your wine happy. The first rule of wine storage is to keep it out of the sun. The second rule is to keep it away from the heat. Avoiding direct sunlight is pretty much self-explanatory when picking a location, but heat can be a little trickier. All you need to do is remember your early science classes…heat rises. Even if the wine isn't directly over the stove, rooms are naturally hotter the closer one is to the ceiling. Also, storing wine out of direct sunlight but along a wall that gets full sunlight can cause warmer conditions along the inside wall of a building.

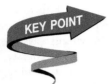

Wine should be stored on its side in a cool, dark environment.

What's the ideal location for your growing wine collection then? For no-fuss ambient (room temperature) storage, you'll want to locate your wine low and in a dark interior location. Of course, cellars and basements are the best, but not everyone has one. Closets without exterior walls work extremely well, as do cabinets that are away from appliances that create heat.

Wine bottles should always be stored on their side (horizontally) to keep the cork moist, thus avoiding it spoiling and damaging the wine.

Author's Aside

There may come a time when you amass a large number of bottles that mark the beginning of a wine collection. If you have a case or two worth of bottles, it is fine to simply use the wine case box as a wine holder. (Most large wine stores and grocery stores will supply you will a case or two for free, if you ask.) When you get more than that, you'll probably want to entertain the purchase of a wine rack. It doesn't have to be a fancy one. In fact, my first wine rack (when I got 28 bottles of wine…most of which was grocery store wine) was a find at a local thrift store.

Beware when the wine bug hits. I quickly outgrew that wobbly wooden one which held 30 bottles. Within a year, I found a metal wine rack with large shelves that could accommodate three rows of bottles on each shelf.

Then came the "all in" moment. I finally got to the point that I insulated a closet (it has an exterior wall), punched a hole in the wall, and added a full-fledged wine refrigeration unit. Yes, the bug hit big. I'd suggest putting off a wine closet, given you have the space, until the cost of a refrigeration unit is 25% or less of the total amount of your wine purchases in a year. That's just a helpful hint for those interested in wine and who have overachiever tendencies with a wine-friendly budget.

THE TAKEAWAY

Wine tools come in a variety of shapes, sizes, and functions. Some are useful "must have" items even for the true beginner. Others are nice to have, and still many items become necessary only after you've developed a regular wine habit. **Here's your chapter cheat sheet:**

▶ The winged corkscrew is the most common corkscrew.

▶ The sommelier knife or wine key is the second most common corkscrew and requires a little more practice to use.

▶ Specialized corkscrews and wine openers are available to assist those who otherwise have difficulty uncorking a bottle.

▶ Decanting wine is the process of pouring a bottle of wine into a large container before serving in a wine glass. This allows the wine to breathe and lets sediment settle before pouring.

▶ Wine glasses come in a variety of shapes and sizes to maximize the tasting experience of a particular type or style of wine.

▶ Wine should never be left in a hot car.

▶ A partial bottle of sparkling wine should only be recorked with a topper designed specifically for sparkling wines.

▶ Wine should be stored on its side in a cool, dark environment.

*"My dear girl, there are some things
that are just not done,
such as drinking Dom Perignon '53
above the temperature of 38° Fahrenheit."*

—James Bond in Ian Fleming's Goldfinger

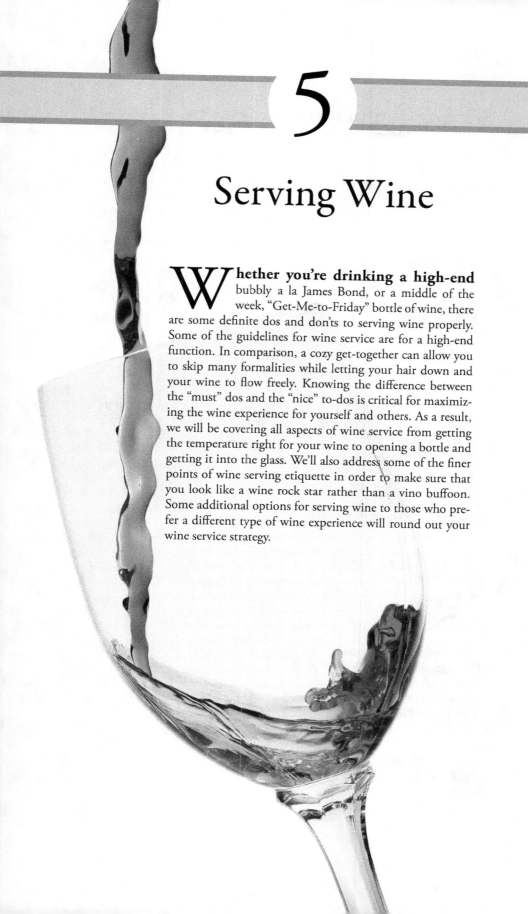

5

Serving Wine

Whether you're drinking a high-end bubbly a la James Bond, or a middle of the week, "Get-Me-to-Friday" bottle of wine, there are some definite dos and don'ts to serving wine properly. Some of the guidelines for wine service are for a high-end function. In comparison, a cozy get-together can allow you to skip many formalities while letting your hair down and your wine to flow freely. Knowing the difference between the "must" dos and the "nice" to-dos is critical for maximizing the wine experience for yourself and others. As a result, we will be covering all aspects of wine service from getting the temperature right for your wine to opening a bottle and getting it into the glass. We'll also address some of the finer points of wine serving etiquette in order to make sure that you look like a wine rock star rather than a vino buffoon. Some additional options for serving wine to those who prefer a different type of wine experience will round out your wine service strategy.

Serving Temperatures

Regardless of whether you are drinking wine in a formal or informal setting, getting the temperature right is critical to getting the most enjoyment from your drinking experience. If your wine is not the right temperature, you will likely be disappointed with the taste because the degree to which your wine is chilled impacts the flavor in your mouth. With that in mind, the ideal temperature for different wines is more a guideline than a hard and fast rule. It is okay to be in the general ballpark with regard to the degree of chill. A few degrees warmer or cooler will not ruin your overall experience.

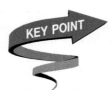

Wine should be served with a degree of chill based on the type and style.

The simplest guideline for knowing what level of chill is best for the wine you are serving is to understand the basic spectrum. The coldest of cold is reserved for sparkling wines. Typically, you want to aim for a range of 38 to 50 degrees for bubblies. This can be considered "freezer cold." For higher-end sparkling wines, you'll want to have them served at the warmer end of that range to allow more of the aroma to be present in the drinking experience. Less expensive (lower or mid-range quality) bubblies should be served colder because the aromas are not as defined.

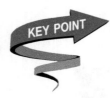

Sparkling wines should be served "freezer cold."

You don't need an expensive wine chiller. An easy and inexpensive guideline for chilling your high-end bubbly to perfection is to let the bottle sit in the freezer for an hour prior to opening it. Mid-range sparkling wines should sit in the freezer for an hour and a half, and lower quality bottles should be in the freezer for a minimum of two hours.

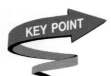

Bottles can be cooled in the freezer for 30 minutes to 2 hours.

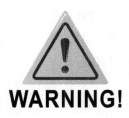

WARNING!

Do not leave any wine bottle in the freezer for an extended period of time (like overnight or longer). The wine will expand and blow the cork out of the bottle. Even the best of us can forget a bottle in the freezer and hear the dreaded bang of the cork letting loose from within it. While the freezer will contain the damage, there is a danger of injury from a cork being expelled when the freezer is open. There is also the possibility that the bottle can be damaged when an explosion happens, causing pieces of glass to shatter everywhere.

The next level of chill covers still, white wines from Pinot Grigios to Chardonnays. These wines should be served slightly warmer than sparkling wines, with a temperature range of between 44 degrees and 57 degrees. Again, there's a general "sub-rule" within that range. The lighter, more acidic the wine is, the cooler it should be. A Pinot Grigio should be served at the lower end of the temperature range. Chardonnays are usually more complex in aroma and bouquet and are best warmer but still within this range. This is especially true for Chardonnays that are more "oaky" in nature. The exception to the general rule here relates to late harvest and dessert white wines. They benefit from being at the cooler temperatures due to the fact that they are high in residual sugars and are served in noticeably smaller portions.

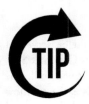

To chill a bottle even faster, wrap it in a wet towel before putting it in the freezer.

To chill your bottle of white wine quickly to "refrigerator cold," you will use a combination of the freezer and the fridge. You can achieve the right white temperature by putting the bottle in the freezer for a half an hour and then placing it in the refrigerator to maintain the chill. If you have the time, you can skip the freezer step and chill the bottle in the fridge for two hours or more. The upper end of the temperature spectrum is achieved by placing the bottle in the refrigerator (not the freezer), for at least an hour prior to serving, and leaving it there to maintain the chill.

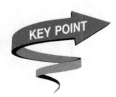

White wines should be served "refrigerator cold."

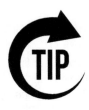

It is easier to allow a wine to warm up than it is to chill it down, so err on the side of a colder bottle and let the wine warm to a preferred temperature in the glass once it is served.

Now, we move from whites to reds. Lighter reds are best served chilled but not cold. I call it "refrigerator cooled" as opposed to cold. The reds in this category include Pinot Noir, and Zinfandels that are less complex. Rosés can be served either fridge cold or fridge cooled depending on your preferences. The temperature range to shoot for with this group of wines is between 53 degrees and 63 degrees. Again, the lighter the wine, the lower in the temperature should be within the given range, so a Rosé will be served around 53 degrees while a fruiter Zinfandel will be best in the low 60s.

Chilling these wines is easy. To achieve the cooled wine bottle for these wines, the best cooling option is to let the bottle sit in the refrigerator for about a half hour before serving.

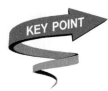 *Light red wines should be served "refrigerator cooled."*

Finally, the conventional wisdom is that red wines should be served at room temperature. The reality is that bolder red wines such as Cabernet Sauvignon, Merlot, or Syrah are best experienced with a little hint of a chill. The ideal temperature is between 63 and 69 degrees. Again, it is easier to allow a wine to warm up, so chilling the wine in a refrigerator for a half hour and then allowing it to remain on the table or counter is the easiest way to regulate the temperature of your bolder red wines.

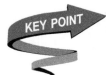 *Bolder red wines should be served slightly below room temperature.*

Here's a quick and easy guide to getting your wines to the most beneficial serving temperatures.

Wine Temperature Cheat Sheet

Sparkling Wines	White Wines	Light Reds	Bold Reds
"Freezer Cold"	"Refrigerator Cold"	"Refrigerator Cooled"	"Chilled"
Temp: 38°— 50°	Temp: 44°— 57°	Temp: 53°— 63°	Temp: 63°— 69°
Chill: Freezer 1 to 2 Hours	**Chill:** Freezer 30 Mins./Leave in Fridge or 2⁺ Hours in Fridge Only	**Chill:** Fridge 30 Mins.	**Chill:** Fridge 30 Mins./Leave on Counter or Table

The more complex the wine is for each category, the higher the serving temperature in the given range.

Now, with all of the talk about the importance of temperature in regard to a top-quality tasting experience, it is important to remember that your wine does not have to be an exact temperature to be enjoyed. These are general guidelines for optimal taste in serving wine. Unless you are an extremely particular engineer or rocket scientist type, it's not necessary to have a thermometer at the ready to decide when to drink your wine. If you happen to have those compulsive tendencies, there are a range of devices that allow you to establish the temperature of a wine bottle without any doubts. Thermometers are available that wrap a bottle in a sleeve to give a temperature reading, if you're so inclined. Personally, I ballpark it, make adjustments as necessary, and do just fine. As with just about everything about wine, your personal preferences will also factor in to the temperature that you enjoy most. No one is going to show up and put handcuffs on you if you prefer your Chardonnay closer to room temperature, or whatever the case may be.

TIP If you find that the wine feels like it is burning your mouth because of an intense alcohol effect in the aroma or on the tongue, you may want to chill your wine further. Conversely, if you are disappointed with the level of flavor in your wine glass, allow it to warm a bit and see if the aroma becomes more apparent.

Opening Wine Bottles

Opening a bottle of wine can be viewed in one of two ways: a necessary means to an end or a part of the overall wine show experience. There are also two types of bottle opening scenarios to master: one for sparkling wines and the other for still wines. Occasionally, a minor wine catastrophe can happen, even to the best of us, that leads to a little more of a challenge in getting the wine from bottle to glass, but you'll be prepared to head off a crisis with a few tips and pointers once you complete this section.

Opening Bubbly Bottles

By far, the most daunting part of wine culture for the beginner is mastering the technique for opening a bottle of sparkling wine. It can indeed be dangerous if it is not done properly. That's not an understatement. However, with some basic rules of the road, you can quickly, easily, and safely open sparkling wine bottles to all your heart's content.

Special Feature...

Faster Than a Speeding Bullet?

Ever wonder how fast the cork from a bottle of bubbly travels? I did, and found some interesting information. While the bullet still travels faster than the cork, it's interesting to find that the scientific folk among us have actually documented the speed at which a cork travels. According to study done in Germany, a cork from a shaken sparkling wine bottle travels at the rate of more than 24 mph.

Temperature impacts not only the taste of wine but also the pressure inside a bottle of bubbly. The scientists also estimated the speed that a cork from a sparkling wine bottle, which is not shaken but instead left in the sun to heat up, could travel. Theoretically, they proved a cork from warmer bubbly could reach a speed of 62 mph when expelled! All the more reason NOT to leave your wine in a car, shake that bubbly up, or point the bottle at anyone while opening it.

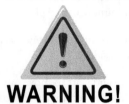

WARNING!

Never, under any circumstances, point the top of a sparkling wine bottle at a person while you are opening it. A cork that flies from a bottle can cause injury or damage to people and objects that are several feet away.

Opening a bottle of sparkling wine can become quite easy to do. You'll want to have a hand towel at the ready before you pop the cork. Let's break it down.

- The first step is to make sure that the bottle is properly chilled. While the cork may expel slightly faster if the bottle is warmer, the trick to enjoying bubbly is to drink it while it is at its freshest and coldest.

- When you are ready to open the bottle, remove the foil and the wire cage. Do not remove the wire cage until you are ready to open the bottle because the pressure will slowly force the cork out of the bottle without assistance if you allow it to sit without the cage. The wire cage is removed taking the loop resting on or near the neck of the bottle and twisting in a counterclockwise direction until the wire is loosened from the cork.

- Now, you will grip the body of the wine bottle in your hand. Some suggest that the bottle be held by your dominant hand, but I use my dominant hand for popping the cork. Do what works best for you by providing the most solid grip.

- Place the bottom of the bottle against your stomach or hip, pointed away from anyone.

- Drape the hand towel on your other arm and place your thumb, going upward, at a 45 degree angle to the bottle.

- Slightly nudge the cork in an upward angle towards the middle of the cork until it begins to dislodge.

TIP

If you have trouble getting the cork to dislodge, you may want to try rubbing the towel on the neck of the bottle. Supposedly, it can help warm the air behind the cork and allow for easier opening. I'm not so sure that a little friction makes that much of a difference on a cold bottle, but it's worth a shot.

- When the cork begins to move slightly, place the towel over the cork and hand you are using to pop the cork, if you wish to minimize any spilling.

- Wrap your opening hand around the cork as you continue to slowly ease the cork from the bottle by rocking the bottle side to side.

- The cork should gain momentum from the pressure and start to move out as you work to open the bottle. As the cork nears its pop, you may want to place your palm over it to slow the ejection.

Contrary to popular belief, bubbly should be opened with a slow, relatively quiet hiss of gas being released and not an explosion. As I was taught when I started opening bubbly, the goal for the sound of bubbly being opened should be similar to the sound of a "nun passing gas in mass." Hilarious, but true.

Special Feature...

En Garde, Bubbly!

Bubbly is a drink associated with celebrations, pomp, and circumstance, so it is fitting that there be a dramatic way of opening sparkling wines. Sabrage is a ceremonial method for opening a bottle of sparkling wine using a saber, sword, knife, or other related instrument. The basic premise is that the sabre breaks away the mouth of the bottle leaving the bubbly flowing freely from the neck and base. The glass from the mouth of the bottle will still be around the cork as the bottle separates, and it makes an interesting wine souvenir for some.

This process is a tradition that is believed to have started with Napoleon, who celebrated with champagne in both victory and defeat. Personally, I think it sounds like a bit of overcompensation by the small-statured French leader, but it does make a good show. Recently, it was a featured element in Cameron Diaz's character in the film *What Happens in Vegas*.

I'm not one to advocate combining sharp objects and alcohol, so I am going to refrain from giving specifics on the technique in the interest of public safety. If you are interested in learning more, in theory of course, that research is up to you.

Opening Still Wines

By comparison, opening a bottle of still wine is simpler than that of a bubbly bottle, and I'm not referencing twist-off tops, either. Screw tops are pretty much self-explanatory, so I'll leave those to you. Now, it's all about the cork. The most common forms of corkscrews are the winged corkscrew and the sommelier's knife, so we'll focus on those to start.

Using a Winged Corkscrew

A winged corkscrew is the most common and often the cheapest form of wine opener. When opening a bottle of wine with a winged corkscrew you will need to use a foil cutter, knife, or the point of the corkscrew to start the foil tear. Let's begin.

- Remove the foil from the bottle using a foil cutter or simply start a tear in the foil with a steak knife or scissors.

- Once the foil is off the bottle, center the point of the corkscrew at the top of the cork.

- Twist the corkscrew down into the cork as far as possible while allowing the arms on either side of the opener to rise up as you go.

- Once the opener is fully twisted into the cork, place the bottle on a flat surface and grab an arm in each hand.

- Press down gently, allowing the cork to be pulled out of the bottle.

Chances are the cork will not be completely freed once the arms are down completely, but a little tug will dislodge the cork from the bottle. Voilà! It's that simple.

Using a Sommelier's Knife

A sommelier's knife takes a little more skill than a winged corkscrew, but not much. This tool is more typical of wine snob pomp and circumstance, but it's easier than you'd think.

- Begin by sliding the foil cutter out of the side. It's the piece that looks like a little pocket knife. Use the cutter to slice off the foil. (It's your personal preference as to whether you circle the top lip of the foil and leave the rest on the neck, or remove the foil completely.)

- Slide the cutter back into place and pull out the leverage arm first. That's the piece that is typically on top of the corkscrew and has a notch on it that will rest on the lip of the bottle.

- Now, pull out the corkscrew arm, locking it in a 90 degree angle from the body of the opener. The key will have a T shape at this point.

- Place the end of the corkscrew in the middle of the cork and twist it into the bottle as far as you can.

- Bend the body of the opener so that the notch of the leverage arm is resting on the lip of the bottle. When the corkscrew is turned into the cork, the side with the leverage arm will be higher than the other one.

- Pull on the opposite end of the opener (the lower one) to begin to dislodge the cork. Again, an extra tug on your part may be necessary to fully remove the cork from the bottle. That's it. You can twist the cork off of the corkscrew and put it away or open to your heart's content.

Crumbling Corks

Though someone relatively new to wine won't often encounter the problem of a cork that disintegrates during the opening process, it's still good to know how to save a stubborn wine bottle. Plus, you may get to be a hero to your fellow wine drinkers after rescuing a bottle.

First of all, cork problems are generally the result of two issues. If the bottle is relatively young, it may be simply a case of a bad cork. Cork is indeed a natural product and sometimes there are inherent problems with the material. If your "problem child" wine falls into this category, it is especially important to be on the lookout for signs of spoilage. Any "off" smell or taste should be taken as a sign of surrender, and the wine should be set aside. In the case of an older wine, say one that is 10 years-plus or stored questionably, the cork may have simply gotten too moist and started to disintegrate. You'll still need to be on the lookout for the wine being "corked" (smelling or tasting like cork), but cork trouble in an older wine is not quite the same red flag as it is in a younger bottle.

There are some special tools that can help with corks that have gotten stuck in the bottle. Quite frankly, unless you regularly drink older bottles or are starting to develop a serious wine collecting habit, these tools may collect more dust than they will be of use. Wine snobs will cringe at the following advice, but I also understand that it's not always handy to run to a store to seek out special tools for getting a cork out of bottle that's in trouble.

Barring any special devices that you may have on hand to handle your wine crisis, there are ways to still get your captive wine from the bottle to the glass. You'll know that you have exhausted your options for using a regular corkscrew when the remaining cork plug is deeper into the neck of the bottle than the extended corkscrew can reach. Stop, take a breath and then clear the bottle neck of as much of the cork particles as you can. You're about to go "Wine MacGyver" mode here. You'll need to grab a long-handled spoon, knife, skewer, or something similar that you have on hand. (I have a set of BBQ skewers that have come in handy for this purpose.) If you have a tea strainer, infuser, or filter, use it to help you minimize the cork shrapnel that makes it to the glass. You'll also need a pitcher or decanter.

Here's where the wine elite scream—push the cork into the wine. Yep, you're going to intentionally sink it. Be careful! The force of the cork hitting the wine will cause splash back. Be as gentle as possible to avoid wearing your wine or having to wipe down the table. (Ask me how I know.)

Once the cork is floating in the wine, you are going to slowly pour the wine from the bottle into your pitcher or decanter. The point here is to be gentle enough to avoid transferring too much cork when you pour. The cork may block the neck, so it will become a balancing act of using your skewer (or knife, etc.) to hold the cork away from the mouth of the bottle while pouring. If that's not enough to stop cork escapees, you'll pour the wine through a straining device, if you have one. I know it sounds complicated and like you need three hands, but I assure you I have used the technique many times. It won't get the fine pieces of cork completely out of your wine, but it will salvage the bottle.

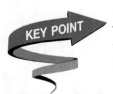

A crumbling cork doesn't mean the wine is automatically ruined, though it can indicate the wine may have a problem from the faulty cork.

Decanting Wine

If you successfully opened your wine with or without a cork crisis, you'll want to consider decanting your wine before serving. This is more important for red wines than white wines, though whites do benefit from a little breathing time. As a quick review from the previous discussion regarding decanters in the Wine Tools section, the process of decanting a wine is also known as letting a wine breathe. While it may sound snobbish, there is a sound rationale for letting wine open up before drinking it. Have you ever opened a bottle of wine and drank it immediately, only to be overpowered by the alcohol in it? Breathing allows that alcohol overload to mellow out in both the aroma and the taste. By allowing the wine to breathe and open up, you allow the fruit in the wine to come forward. Plus, if you are drinking an unfiltered wine or an older wine that has sediment in the bottle, it allows the sediment to settle somewhere other than in your glass.

It sounds like a special process, but in reality decanting is probably the simplest step in the wine consumption experience, even easier than drinking it. Seriously. To decant a wine, open the bottle ahead of time and pour it into a decanter, pitcher, or similar container. Then, ignore it. I said it was the simplest step, not necessarily easiest. Yes, it's tempting to start drinking the grapey goodness once the cork's been popped, but decanting is a pour-and-wait game. Patience, unfortunately, is a virtue here.

The length of time that you let the wine sit can depend on several factors. Reds will need to breathe longer than whites. Wines with sediment will need to rest until they clear up as the particles collect at the bottom of the decanter. Typically, you'll want to allow the wine to breathe at least an hour before drinking to allow it to completely open up. Some bold and highly tannic wines may need even longer.

If you don't have a decanter or pitcher, you can still get some benefit from letting an open wine bottle sit. You'll be able to get to your wine a little quicker if you pour some into glasses to let it contact the air more than it would in the bottle. There are pocket aerators that can also speed up the process without a decanter. They look like a special kind of sieve that you hold over a glass and pour the wine through. It's not the same as decanting and a little patience, but it does help while giving you something to talk about within a wine crowd.

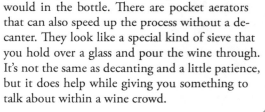

Author's Aside

If you're still not convinced that letting your wine breathe makes the wine taste better, I dare you to try this challenge. It involves drinking two bottles of wine (a sacrifice, I know). The next time you're at the store, buy two bottles of the exact the same wine. It is best if it is a bolder red wine or red blend. When you are ready for the challenge, open and decant one bottle for at least one hour, preferably 90 minutes. When you're ready to drink, pour a glass of the decanted wine. When you're done with the first glass, open the other bottle and immediately drink a glass from the "fresh" bottle. You'll experience, firsthand, the difference between a wine that has opened up and one that has not.

Pouring Wine ——————

You may be asking, "Geez already, can we get the wine in the glass now?" The answer is yes!

Of course, there are some finer points to understand even here. I know here are a few eye rolls in the crowd, but bear with me. Here, the considerations are focused on the glasses to use, the amount to pour, and the order to pour in for times when multiple wines are served.

When it comes to the proper glass in which to serve wine, the first consideration is what you have on hand. If you don't have wine glasses and need to use another type of glass, so be it. Enjoy your wine, and return to this part of the discussion when you have wine glasses. No harm, no foul. If you have a selection of wine glasses, the general rule is that sparkling wines should be served in flutes of some type. The distinction between red and white wine glasses is more important for those who have developed a wine habit. If you have different sizes of the more traditional wine glass shapes, the rule is that glasses with a smaller rim are best for whites while bigger bowls and rims are suited more for reds.

The order in which wines should be served is based on maximizing the experience of each type and varietal of wine. Personal preference will always trump the "shoulds" of wine service. If someone wants to skip to the bold reds, be a good host and oblige. Otherwise, the general approach to wine service is sparkling wine first. In some cases, it may be served last as part of a separate dessert service though. Then, you want to think light to dark, first for white then the same for reds. Dessert wines are last if they are being served.

Wines should be served by starting with sparkling wine, if it is to be served as part of a meal or gathering, because it can be overpowered by some of even the lightest white still wines. Once the bubbly has been consumed, then follow through the whites, starting with the lightest and driest first. When moving into red wines, follow the same pattern as the whites. When deciding between two or three bottles at a gathering the following points should help:

- Light wines are to be served before full-bodied wines (generally whites before reds);
- Drier wines are to be served before sweeter wines;
- Lesser-quality wines are to be served before higher-quality wines; and
- When it comes to red wines, younger vintages are to be served before older vintages.

These guidelines will see you through any dinner or function where you will be serving wine. However, a discussion in the section will cover larger wine flights that are served during wine tastings and will explore varietal-specific lineups.

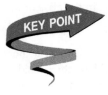

When deciding which bottle to serve first, follow the general guidelines: sparkling wines first; lighter before darker (whites before reds); drier before sweeter; lower quality before higher quality; younger vintages before older vintages (especially for red wines).

In practical terms, the amount of wine poured into the glass depends on the circumstances. If it's an informal gathering or a TGIF moment, the pours will usually be greater. For more formal functions, the typical serving is 3-4 ounces until everyone who wants a drink is served. Once everyone has had a chance to partake, pours can go to the standard 6-8 ounce pours while wine remains. It's simply about courtesy. The other reason to use this method of pouring is to be able to rein in would-be wine hogs more easily. After all, it is important to remember that wine bottles are not bottomless. If you pour 4 ounces per glass, you should be able to serve about six people. If you pour 6-8 ounce glasses, that number drops to between 3 and 4 glass per bottle. Just keep that in mind when selecting the number of bottles you will be serving.

An easy way to gauge a pour without looking like a wine miser and measuring is to allow the wine to flow up to the widest part of the glass. Aside from a method of measuring pours, this level in the glass is another way to help the wine breathe by giving it the greatest amount of surface contact with the air. Now, you can regulate the amount of wine in each glass while sounding like a true wine aficionado and not a cost-conscious host.

Service Etiquette Basics

While I don't embarrass myself or others in public, I'll be the first to admit that I've never read *Miss Manners* either. With that in mind, there are a few pointers in the area of wine service manners that are required reading for anyone who is serving wine. I'll keep it brief and to the point, giving you just enough to allow you to rest assured that you will look like a hero rather than a villain during any of your wine service duties. These pointers are designed for smaller situations like dinners. For tips about larger wine tasting parties, be sure to review the next section to insure you have a smooth-running event.

Rules for Great Wine Hosting

Be Prepared: When hosting a wine-fueled gathering, have your wines ready to go before your guests arrive. Remember it is about your guests and not all about you. Even if you drink only red wines, have at least one bottle of white wine chilled and ready to serve when guests arrive. There's nothing worse than having guests (or their companions) arrive and make a request for a glass of white wine that tastes bad because you had to serve it at room temperature. Similarly, make sure that you have enough clean glasses beforehand to cover the number of guests that you expect. Wine is served at more formal gatherings through a one-on-one pour. For informal gatherings, glasses can be set out on a table or counter to encourage guests to pour at their leisure. Also, have glasses for water, bottled water, and other non-alcoholic beverages available for guests throughout your gathering.

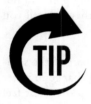 You may want to chill flutes and white wine glasses before your gathering, in a manner similar to serving beer in a frosted mug. It will help keep the wine cooler longer.

Offer, Don't Wait: As the host of a dinner or gathering involving wine, be sure that you offer you guests a glass of wine upon arrival. Guests should be served first. Even if you start sipping before guest arrive, immediately offer them a glass when they are greeted. Do not wait for them to request a drink.

Ladies and Experience First: When pouring wine at the table or for a group at a set time, serve the ladies first, followed by older guests and VIPs. The logic is that this is based on polite behavior. (Who said that chivalry is dead?) Once the ladies have been served, offer wine to those who are older. Again, this is a sign of respect. Plus, women and older guests will likely curb their consumption first (not always, but as a general observation). If there is a VIP guest who hasn't been served already, they will likely go next, followed by those who have not been otherwise served. Sorry, fellas.

Host First, Drink Second: When it comes time to refill glasses, offer a re-pour to your guests' glasses before refilling your own. This is more important for a sit-down affair where everyone is gathered in one location than it is for an informal, mingling event. For the more relaxed setting, offer to refill the glasses of those around you before pouring your own. You don't need to check every glass at an informal party every time that you want to refill.

Keep Wine in Reach: During the course of a meal that is served with wine, allow your guests access to bottles in order to show your hospitality. You can expect guests to drink between a half and full bottle of wine, each, when a meal is served. In addition to having enough wine to cover your guests drinking needs, place open wine bottles or decanters within reach for those choosing to partake. A rule of thumb is to have one or two bottles at the table for a party of four. Add a bottle to the table for every additional 2-4 people and place the bottles throughout the table.

Good to the Last Drop: When you reach the end of a bottle, offer the remaining wine to guests first, and then pour it for yourself if there are no takers. There's no need to be a rude wine miser.

Ask about Gift Bottles: If you have an unopened bottle of wine that a guest brought to the gathering, you should offer the bottle back to the guest to take home at the end of the night. Do not assume a guest wants to subsidize your wine collection when they simply were being polite in not showing up empty handed. If they meant it to be a gift, they will tell you to keep it anyway.

Handling the Tipsy: If a guest has had too much, be part of the solution. To slow down a power drinker, lead by example and change to water or another beverage and offer one to the guest. It will help the guest feel like they aren't the only one without a drink in hand. Later in the evening, you can also begin to clear the table or counter of wine to slow down everyone's drinking in a non-confrontational way. At the end of the night, allow your guests time to let the effects of wine clear before venturing out. If it becomes late and a guest is still tipsy, offer to call a cab, arrange another ride, or a crash out in a guest room or on the couch. The point is that you want your gathering to be a pleasant and safe event from start to finish, and the finish includes guests returning home safely.

Author's Aside

Depending on those who join you for a wine dinner or gathering, you may get unexpected requests. Remember that the point is for everyone to have an enjoyable wine experience. While a wine snob will wrinkle their nose at the idea of adding ice to a glass of wine or watering it down with soda, the guest is always right. You are not responsible for nor are you the dictator of other people's preferences. You may want to ask if they would like the wine chilled more if they ask for ice in their wine glass. It may be that simple. In other circumstances, it may be that having ice or soda in their wine is the only way they have ever consumed wine. Make them happy – you can enjoy your wine your way.

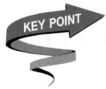

KEY POINT *Proper etiquette includes: host first/drink second; ladies first followed by older and honored guests; keep wine within reach for dinner service with multiple bottles if necessary; and offer guests the last sip of wine from a bottle before pouring it for yourself.*

Additional Wine Options

Consider this a special bonus section to your wine service knowledge. There will be times when either you or a guest would prefer to drink something other than a glass of pure wine. There are some wine-based drink options that can extend the life of your party or gathering to those who have a hankering for something a little different from the usual wine fare.

MIMOSAS

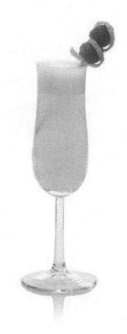

For those who would like bubbly, but do not necessarily want a full glass, mimosas are a refreshing option. Mimosas are popular for brunches and daytime functions by lightening up the alcohol content in each glass. Though mimosas can be served in flutes like full glasses of sparkling wine, often it is best to use a full-size red wine glass for the quick and easy bubbly change-up.

Mimosas are simple. The basic mimosa is a combination of one part bubbly and one part orange juice. If you want to jazz up the basic mimosa, try adding a few mandarin oranges to each drink. Don't be afraid to experiment with other fruit juices. A personal favorite of mine is a combination of orange and mango juice which can be easily found in grocery stores. Mimosas are also a great way to use up any leftover bubbly from a previous night's festivities.

SANGRIA

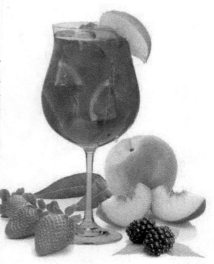

Sangria can be described as a type of "wine punch" that originated in Spain and Portugal. It is comprised of wine, fruit, and a sweetener such as fruit juice, soda, or sugar/honey. There are both red and white sangria options based on the wine used. The drink is a wonderful party option and is a refreshing drink for gatherings in warmer weather. The added fruit provides a flavor boost and light snack at the end of each glass. A plethora of sangria recipes exist, and creating your own version is simple. A basic sangria recipe for red or white sangria can lay the foundation for further exploration. You can find my personal recipes in the Deep Dish at the end of the book.

Author's Aside

 I have a friend who is obsessed with Sangria drinks. If you are interested in learning more about the options for sangrias using red, white, and sparkling wines as well as ciders, check out Gina Lynn's books for quick and handy ideas. The first book, Sensational Sangrias, focuses on red and white wine options. Mimosagrias uses sparkling wines for sangria drinks. If you want to walk on the wild side, she has a Cider-gria book that uses pear and apple ciders for sangria like drinks. I've been a sangria lab rat for her work and some of them are both surprising and taste amazing.

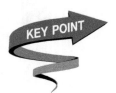

KEY POINT Additional wine options include mimosas and sangria. There are recipes for both (as well as mulled wine) in the Deep Dish at the end of the book.

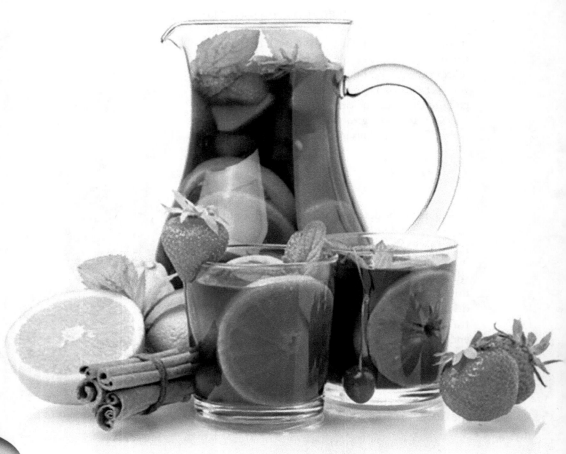

THE TAKEAWAY

Serving wine does not have to be all about special rituals and dramatic flair. In fact, it is a simple process once you are familiar with some basic concepts that ensure that you and your guests have the best tasting experience within a pleasant social setting. **Here are the key points from this chapter:**

► Wine should be served with a degree of chill based on the type and style.

► Sparkling wines should be served "freezer cold."

► White wines should be served "refrigerator cold."

► Light red wines should be served "refrigerator cool."

► Bolder red wines should be served "chilled" slightly below room temperature.

► Bottles can be cooled by being placed in the freezer or refrigerator for 30 minutes to 2 hours.

► Do not leave bottles in the freezer for an extended period of time. Deeper freezing will cause the cork to blow out of the bottle.

► When opening a bottle of sparkling wine, never point the cork at anyone because of the risk of injury.

► A crumbling cork doesn't mean the wine is automatically ruined, though it can indicate the wine may have a problem from the faulty cork.

► When deciding which bottle to serve first follow the general guidelines: sparkling wines first; lighter before darker (whites before reds); drier before sweeter; lower quality before higher quality; younger vintages before older vintages (especially for red wines).

► Proper etiquette includes: host first/drink second; ladies first followed by older and honored guests; keep wine within reach for dinner service with multiple bottles if necessary; and offer guests the last sip of wine from a bottle before pouring it for yourself.

► Additional wine options include mimosas, sangria, and mulled wine.

*"Accept what life offers you and try to drink from every cup.
All wines should be tasted; some should only be sipped,
but with others, drink the whole bottle."*

—Paulo Coelho, *Brida*

6

Wine Tasting

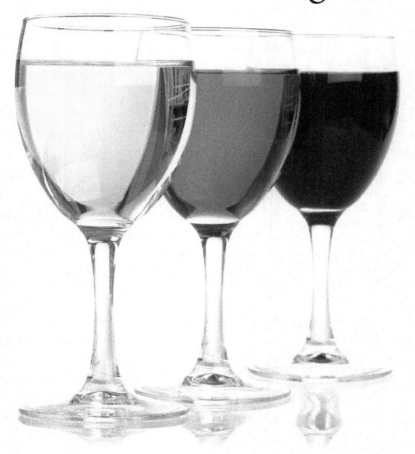

Wine tasting can be divided into categories. The first element includes the mechanics of wine tasting, which includes using more than just your taste buds to evaluate the liquid in your glass. You will learn both the steps to drinking your wine in a manner that allows you to fully enjoy the grapey goodness, as well as the reasons why wine drinkers do what they do. Once you understand the mechanics of tasting wine, the discussion will cover the second category of wine tasting: the social element. This includes wine tasting in the form of parties and winery visits. By the end of the section, you will know how to experience your wines in a manner that allows you to avoid any faux pas.

Wine Tasting Mechanics

The wine tasting process is more than tasting what is in the glass. It is actually a full sensory experience. You will use your sight, smell, taste, and touch most directly. Hearing comes into play if you are doing your tasting with a fellow wine drinker and sharing your observations. The process of wine tasting is comprised of the 5 S's: sight, swirl, smell, sip, and swallow or spit. Each of the steps serves a purpose and is not simply about being snobbish.

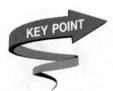

The mechanics of wine tasting are comprised of the 5 S's: sight, swirl, smell, sip, and swallow/spit.

Sight

When you first encounter wine in a glass, it will be through your sense of sight. It is important to look at the wine before you put it to your lips, at least for the first sip. The appearance of the wine can give you information about what to expect from the glass. Similar to the process for shopping for a diamond ring, you are observing the color and clarity of the liquid. The best way to do this is to look at the wine against a white background in a well-lit area. It is one of the reasons that tablecloths are white in finer dining establishments. If you don't have a white tablecloth, a napkin or shirt can work just as well.

You can expect the following color characteristics for wines:

- **Sparkling wines** can range from nearly clear to medium yellow, or pale to rosy pink for bubbly made in contact with the grape skins.

- **White wines** can range from clear or nearly clear to pale greens, all shades of yellow, and gold or honey colors. Colors tend to intensify with age in white wines, though oaked Chardonnays can present with a deeper color at an earlier age.

- **Red wines** can range from a bright red to ruby, burgundy, brick, purple, and even brown. As reds age, the red color tends to degrade from reds to browns.

**Some questions to answer when examining
the appearance of your wine include:**

- **Is the wine clear or cloudy?** A cloudy wine can indicate age, as sediment has developed. Also, the degree of filtering used can be seen. Unfiltered wines will be cloudier.

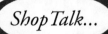

Shop Talk...

18. **Legs**, noun. The little rivulets of wine that trickle down the side of a glass as wine is poured or swirled while coming to a rest in the bowl of the glass. Legs are fun wine phenomena that indicate higher levels of residual sugar in a wine, or a wine that has a higher alcohol content. They are not scientific and are more of a talking point among wine drinkers than an indication of quality.

- **Is it vivid in color, deep in color, or dull?** Brighter colored wines will likely be younger.

- **Is it the same color throughout?** Wine (especially reds) can have a different shade around the edges of the drink rim due to age or the varietals that are blended together.

- **How does the wine flow down the inside of the glass? Is there any lingering film of wine on the sides of the glass?** If the wine appears to have little streams that run down the sides of the glass, these are called "legs." The slower they move and the larger they appear indicates a higher residual sugar level in the wine, or a higher alcohol content.

KEY POINT *When visually examining a wine, look for color and clarity.*

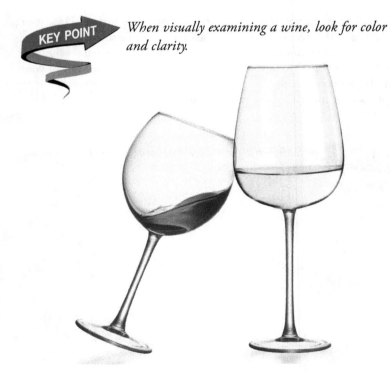

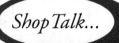

Shop Talk...

19. **Aroma**, noun. The aroma of a wine is the overall smell. Wine drinkers will often use the terms "aroma" and "bouquet" interchangeably though the terms are technically referring to different aspects of smell sensations.

Swirl

This is a transition step between observing the wine and smelling the wine. It serves two purposes. First, it allows the wine's aroma to intensify in the glass as the wine has more contact with the air. This is part of the breathing process as well, but more importantly, this step makes it easier to detect the wine's aroma prior to tasting. Second, if you did not examine the legs of the wine in the previous step, watching the wine settle back into the bowl of the glass will give you an opportunity to observe their nature.

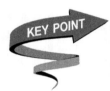

Swirling the wine helps open up the wine to get a better aroma in the glass.

To swirl properly, you should rest the glass on a flat surface. Place your fingers around the stem or base of the glass and swirl in either a clockwise or counter clockwise motion. Unless your goal is to warm up your wine, you should avoid swirling your wine by cupping the bowl of the glass in your palm. As you continue to taste your wine, you can return to swirling it to help it open up more and taste more approachable. This is especially helpful for younger and bolder wines.

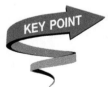

Swirling a glass should be done by the base or stem of the glass, not the bowl.

Aroma versus Bouquet

You will often hear the term "bouquet" for the smell of a wine in a glass. Some will use the term "aroma" instead. Are they interchangeable, or will you look like a fool for using one rather than the other? Technically, there is a difference between the use of the two terms. Aroma is an overall smell profile. It can be divided into categories based on the characteristics experienced from the glass. Aroma is most strictly associated with the varietal and vinous characteristics. Varietal aromas are tied to the grape used (i.e. Zinfandel versus Cabernet Sauvignon) and are present in all wines of the given varietal. For Zinfandels, it could be the "jamminess" of the wine versus the licorice of a Cabernet Sauvignon. Vinous aromas are smells that result from the growth and fermentation of a wine. These would include influences of the land (terroir) and elements within the growing environment. The third category for aromas is really what is referred to when discussing bouquet. Therefore, a wine's bouquet is technically a sub-class of the wine's aroma. The bouquet is comprised of tertiary aromas that are the result of aging and the fermentation process. The most notable of these aromas will be the presence of an oak smell or any of the associated characteristics regarding aging in an oak barrel or steel cask. Compare the smell of an oaked Chardonnay to one done in steel for the easiest way to differentiate bouquets.

Will anyone look at you and shake their head sadly if you refer to the general aroma of a wine as the bouquet? Probably not, unless you are with the seriously wine elite. Even the pros mischaracterize the aroma as the bouquet from time to time.

137

Smell

The smell of the wine does indeed influence the taste of it. Taste is actually a combination of smell and taste. No two people will experience the aroma of a wine in the same way. This is for a variety of reasons. There are dozens, if not hundreds, of aromas in wine. If you have a cold or an allergy with a stuffy nose, you may not be able to pick up on the more subtle scents. Experience plays a role in how you process aromas as well. If you are not familiar with a specific aroma, say currants or lychee fruit, you may not be able to detect it or name it, if you do smell it. More experienced wine drinkers will pick up aromas that someone new to wine will not. Just because you smell something that someone else does not, or vice versa, does not mean that either of you is wrong.

Because of the variations in wine aroma, it is perfectly acceptable to smell your wine deeply and multiple times. There's no shame in really sticking your nose down into the glass to get the full sensory experience. Taking a big whiff is encouraged among wine lovers. It's not like slurping your soup, so take in all that you can. Don't be afraid to repeatedly sniff your wine as you drink it either. Often you will pick up new aromas as you continue to taste the wine and it opens up more in your glass.

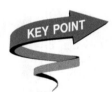 *It is completely acceptable to stick your nose into a glass and inhale deeply.*

You can expect the following aromas in wines:

- **Fruits of all types** are common in wine. After all, wine is made from grapes. There are other fruits that are present in different varietals though. White wines may have apple, citrus, peach, apricot, melon, or tropical fruits. Reds may have berries, currants, plum, and cherry among its fruiter notes.

- **Herbs and spices** are often noted in the aroma of wines. White wines, such as Rieslings and Gewürztraminers, will have elements of cloves and cinnamon. Red wines may have aromas of cocoa, pepper, and anise.

- **Floral notes** are also part of wine aroma. White wines may have hints of rose, lavender, honeysuckle, and even grass (though technically not a floral smell). Red wines can have smells of lavender and violet.

- **Earthy notes** can be found in wines as well because of the influence of the growing environment and the fermentation process. Notice that I did not say a "dirt" taste, but that may be the first word that comes to mind with these aromas. White wines and red wines can have a stone or gravely smell at times. Influences of wood, smoke, tobacco, and tea are also common in red wine varietals.

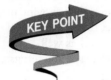

The aroma will have a variety of characteristics, including fruit, herb, spice, floral, and earthy notes.

Some questions to answer when evaluating the smell of your wine:

- **What's the first thing that you smell in the wine? Does it have a single aroma that is more powerful than others?**

- **What other characteristics do you smell? If fruit is the first thing you smell, does another aroma from a different type of smell come to your nose once you process the aroma? Are they what you would expect or are they more unusual?**

Shop Talk…

20. **Nose**, noun. The "wine speak" term for the aroma of a wine. Though the term is used in the context of phrasing such as "The nose of the wine is…" it is really referring to what the taster experiences when smelling and evaluating a wine.

- **Is there a lot of alcohol in the aroma?** Younger wines will tend to have a greater aroma of alcohol. If you are overpowered by an alcohol haze as you inhale, you may need to let the wine breathe longer to fully enjoy it.

- **Are there any "off" smells?** Certain smells can indicate flaws with your wine. A musty or cork smell could indicate a damaged cork has tainted the wine. Other smells that can mean that your wine has a problem include vinegar, chemical smells similar to nail polish remover or Easter egg dyes, sulfur (think rotten eggs), or a sherry smell that may be like burnt marsh-mallows. Other smells that may be signs of problems are barnyard-like aromas and even a nose on the wine that is similar to a Band-Aid.

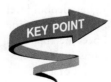

The smell of a wine is the aroma and can be referred to as the nose.

Sip

Now is the really good part. You get to sip your wine. I said sip, not chug. If you are into chugging your wine, I doubt you would have gotten this far into the book, but I had to put it out there. You want just enough wine in your mouth so that you can freely swish it around to get the full impact of it. You want to roll it around on your tongue to get the feel as well as the taste of the wine because different parts of your tongue taste specific things.

KEY POINT *Sipping involves letting the wine roll around in your mouth to get the sensations of taste and texture.*

Wine on the Taste Buds

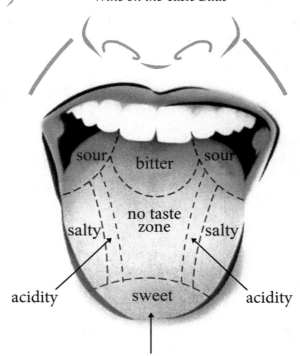

You'll Get the Greatest Sensation at the Tip of Your Tongue!

If you are tasting a sweet wine, you will get the greatest sensation at the tip of your tongue. Highly acidic wines will feel like they light up the middle sides of your tongue. Don't confuse the burn of a higher alcohol level with the acidity of the wine. These are two different things. When the wine hits the back of your tongue, the level of bitterness will become apparent. An element of the bitterness factor is related to the tannins in red wines, which is why reds are often appreciated most towards the end of a sip.

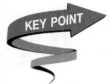

Different areas of the tongue pick up different elements: sweetness (tip), saltiness (outside edge), acidity (inside edge), and bitterness (back).

While you are moving the wine around on your tongue to pick up the flavors, you also want to experience the mouth feel of the wine. The feel of the wine includes sensations of the wine thickness, as well as any sedimentary concerns.

The true nature of taste is a combination of smell and the act of tasting wine. In the strictest sense of the word, taste is limited to the sensations of sweet, salty, acidic, and bitter, combined with the texture of the wine. In real terms, taste is the combination of the aroma and the other sensations to make up the total flavor experience. No one is going to talk about wine without referencing the overall experience.

Questions to answer when evaluating the taste of your wine:

- **Do you like it?** Let's face it, this is priority number one. If you like it, great! If you don't like it, you do not necessarily want to give up on it. You may wait to see if it grows on you as you sip it. The wine may open up more, or simply become more to your liking as you drink more of it. The chill of your wine may need to be adjusted to make it more enjoyable as well. If white wine seems to have no flavor, let it warm a bit. If a red feels like it burns, try chilling it longer before giving up on it. Also, some wines, especially bolder reds, may taste better when sipped with food, so try a nibble of something to balance the wine further. However, if it's just plain bad or you just don't like it at all, there's no need to torture yourself. Find something else that you can enjoy.

- **What are the first sensations that you experience? What are the most noticeable? Is it sweet? Too sweet? Is it acidic to the point that you can't taste anything else?**

- **What flavors do you pick up? Do new flavors emerge as you continue to let it roll on your tongue? What fruity, floral, spicy, and earthy characteristics emerge when you combine your sense of smell and taste? Is any one element more powerful than the others?**

- **How does it feel on your tongue? Is it thick and viscous ("chewy"), or is it flat and thin like water?**

Swallow or Spit

You've got the wine in your mouth. Now you need to decide (if you haven't already) whether to spit it out or swallow it. In the vast majority of situations, you will be tasting wine not just to evaluate it but to enjoy it as well. That makes the decision a no-brainer. If you have a health condition where alcohol consumption needs to be limited or you are going to be tasting many wines in a relatively short time, the best option may be to spit out all or most of your tastings.

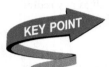

KEY POINT

To spit or to swallow wine is a matter of personal choice and preference.

Author's Aside

The true wine snob will say you must always spit. Hogwash! It's your wine… your experience. You can do as you wish. 99.99% of the time you will be with fellow drinkers rather than spitters.

If you need to spit your wine out in a public setting, there are some steps that you can take to do so in a discreet manner. The least oblivious way to take care of the issue is to pour just enough into your glass for a single sip. Once you are done tasting the wine, simply spit it back into your glass, and then you can empty the glass without making a production out of it. We'll cover more public settings in the coming discussions on wine tastings and winery visits.

Whether you consume or dispose of your tasting wine, there are elements to consider in this phase of your tasting experience. These elements comprise the finish or aftertaste of the wine.

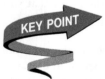

KEY POINT

Once wine has been swallowed or spit out, the wine's aftertaste or finish becomes apparent. A longer finish (30 seconds or more) is desirable for higher quality wines.

You can expect the following in the finish of wines:

• **Bitterness** will not become fully apparent until the wine is swallowed or hits the back of the tongue.

• The **staying power** of wines, especially reds, is part of the experience.

Take your time between sips to see if the impact of the wine lingers in your mouth. The length of the finish can be an indicator of quality for certain varietals.

Questions to answer when evaluating the finish:

- **Does the finish pack a punch?** The finish is where you will experience the tannins in the wine most. Tannins can be described as hard or soft based on the intensity of the bitterness.

- **What is the length of the finish? Is the finish long, short, non-existent?** Lighter white wines will often have a shorter finish, but that is not a universal rule. Both red and white whites can have varying finish lengths.

- **Does the wine seem balanced? Did the finish overwhelm (or underwhelm) the rest of the tasting experience?**

There you have it. These steps make up the basic mechanics of tasting wine. Once you have completed the steps in tasting your wine, you have two options. One, you can move on to a new selection and complete the process again. Two, you can relax and enjoy the rest of your wine by repeating any or all of the steps with the glass before you. The bottom line is there is no right or wrong answer when it comes to what you discover in your wine. As you continue to enjoy wine, your ability to detect more things with regard to the look, smell, and taste of wine will further develop. In this case, practice is the key to greater enjoyment. I know, it's a sacrifice, but the wine gods smile on you for your efforts.

Oh, by the way: in the Deep Dish, at the end of this book, you'll find a Cheat Sheet for 30 Common Wine Tasting Descriptors you can use to navigate your way around the wine experience. It's a nice little summary of this chapter and will help the next time you're exploring a new wine.

Author's Aside

If you find that you are actively developing your wine knowledge and experience, you may want to take notes on your preferences to help with future selections. There is no set way to make wine notes. Some people do scores, stars, or smiley faces. Some note the wine's characteristics. Others will include thoughts about parings or additional serving suggestions. You take the notes, so you make the rules.

Tasting notes do not have to be fancy. I've taken notes on napkins, in note pads, and even on my smartphone. (Yes, there's an app—or two—for that.)

Wine Tasting Parties

Wine is truly a social experience that is best enjoyed with others. A tasting party is one of the most common ways to share in the enjoyment of wine. Like with wine in general, a wine tasting party can be as small or as large and as simple or as complex as you choose it to be. The options are limited only by your goals for the gathering and your creativity. Here, you will learn about a basic format for organizing a wine tasting party, as well as some tips to make it as stress-free as possible.

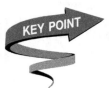

Wine tasting parties can be a fun and relatively easy way to combine learning about wine and socializing.

Planning Your Event

The first thing you will do in planning your wine tasting party is to decide what type of event you want to have. Wine tastings can be done as a stand-alone gathering or combined with a dinner or other element. They can be designed in a manner that highlights a particular theme. Common themes include:

- A dessert tasting that features dessert wines and sweets
- A tasting for a particular type of food (such as BBQ)
- A certain style of wine (such as sparkling, red, or white)
- A geographic sampling with wines from specific regions
- A focus on a specific varietal and selections from various regions
- A particular price point (such as wines under $20)

Once you have established the theme for your tasting, you will want to establish the timing of your event. You'll want to pick a time that allows guests to enjoy the experience, so weekends and holidays are usually the most popular option. Regardless of the date, time, or location for your event, you will need to plan your event with general weather considerations in mind. A hot summer night may not be the best time to host a wine tasting featuring intense red wines, but it may work best for a barbecue tasting in which big reds are paired with food. In that case, you may need to have a selection of chilled whites available, as guests may prefer lighter, cooler wines even with barbecued foods. For events where a meal is to be served, you will also need to decide if you are going to have the meal before or after the tasting—or if folks will taste throughout the event.

Author's Aside

I've been to wine tasting parties with as few as four people and with as many as 50. In my experience, the best parties have between 6 and 12 guests. This allows for one to two bottles of each wine to cover everyone attending the gathering, and the size is intimate enough to encourage conversation between all people. If you are having a tasting with more than a dozen people, you'll want to have an additional bottle of each wine being tasted for every additional 6 people. For example, you should have 4 bottles of each tasting wine for a party with 24 people to be safe.

The next planning issue to address is the extent to which guests will contribute to the event. Will you be providing everything, or are you going to ask guests to bring something? It is common to ask guests to participate in bringing wine or food to a wine tasting, so don't feel awkward about asking. Even if you decide to do everything, don't be surprised if your guests still bring a bottle or snack to the event.

If you want guests to bring items, you will need to do two things to make your tasting party a success. First, you will need to set up a firm RSVP policy. Wine tastings require a hard head count to be sure that you have enough of everything. Second, you will need to be clear about what you want each guest to bring. You should give specific assignments. For example, for a dessert party where you want bubbly, dessert wines, and desserts, you will assign items such as a bottle of late harvest Riesling, a bottle of extra brut bubbly, a tawny Port bottle, a Zinfandel Port bottle, brownies, chocolate chip cookies, spice cake, etc. If you are doing a geographically-themed party, you will want to assign bottles from each targeted region. For example, if you are doing a tasting of Pinot Noir, you will make assignments for a bottle from Oregon, Sonoma, Santa Barbara, Burgundy, etc.

For the simplest and most approachable wine tasting, assign each guest a varietal and let them know that bottles should be under $20. My suggestion is to have a bottle of each of the following: Pinot Grigio, Un-oaked Chardonnay, Oaked Chardonnay, Riesling, Gewürztraminer, Pinot Noir, Merlot, Zinfandel, and Cabernet Sauvignon. All of them are found easily, and the core varietals should make all types of wine drinkers happy. If it is a larger party, and you want sparkling wine to start the party with, you can also assign one or two guests to bring a bottle of bubbly.

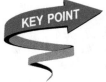

Have one bottle per guest as a general rule. While some will not drink a full bottle during the course of the party, this will ensure that you have enough to cover everyone. Keep a couple extra on hand, as well, in case a guest fails to bring their assigned wine.

As part of your invitation, be sure to make it clear as to what guests can expect. If you are not serving a full meal, let guests know that there will only be a selection of hors d'oeuvres or desserts. Also, let your guests know that they do not necessarily have to break the bank with their choice of wine. It will help take some of the pressure off of guests who may not have a large amount of disposable income.

Ask your guests to avoid wearing heavy perfumes or colognes because strong scents can make tasting wine difficult. There's nothing worse than sitting next to someone who reeks of cologne as you are trying to smell your wine.

Before the day of the tasting party, be sure to do some research on the wines you will be serving. These notes will provide you with material to share with your guests as you introduce the wines. You can present your research notes as trivia items to make the wines more accessible in the minds of your guests and make the tasting a more lively experience.

Preparing for Your Event

Setting up for your wine tasting does not have to be overwhelming. Once you've decided whether your tasting party is going to be a formal sit-down affair (meal or no meal) or a casual mingling event, you will need to establish your serving area. Either way, you should avoid the use of scented candles or flowers that have strong scents in areas where wine tasting will occur. Wine tastings work best if there are one or two central locations for food and drinks. Formal events will likely be centered at a single table, but informal parties flow well if there are separate food and wine tables to avoid having guests crowded together in a limited space.

The supplies that you should have on hand for your wine tasting are as follows:

- **Wine Glasses**:
  You don't need to have a new glass for each glass for each taste. A single red or white glass is sufficient for each guest. If sparkling wine is being served in combination with other wines, you should have a flute available for each guest in addition to a more general wine glass.

- **Water**:
  There should be plenty of water available for guests to drink and to rinse glasses out between tastes. Pitchers are better than bottled water and should be readily accessible to guests. Be sure to have enough water glasses for everyone.

- **Corkscrews and a Foil Cutter**:
  Have at least 2 corkscrews on hand just in case you need a backup or a guest offers to aid in opening bottles. A foil cutter is a cheap wine tool that comes in extremely handy when opening multiple bottles too.

- **Large Bowl**:
  A large container needs to be available for guests to be able to pour out any wine that isn't consumed. Also, it is for the water used to rinse glasses between tastes.

- **Chiller/Ice Bucket**:
  Another large bucket filled approximately halfway with ice and a little water is a way to keep whites and bubbly chilled without having to use the refrigerator.

- **Tablecloth/Napkins**:
  For a table tasting, use a white tablecloth to assist guest in viewing wines. If the party is more about mingling, white napkins can be used for the same purposes while still allowing for the ease of movement.

- **Note-Taking Materials**:
  Paper and writing instruments will allow guests to write out what they think about their tastings without worrying about forgetting anything.

- **Food Items**:
  Even if you are not doing a complete meal, you should have a selection of food available to guests. At the most basic level, you should have snacks within reach that help people clear their palate between tastes. Crackers, cheeses, meats, and such are easy selections. If you are serving Cabernet Sauvignon, you will make your guests smile by having a little chocolate on hand to compliment the wine. Otherwise, your food items will follow your pre-arranged theme and situation.

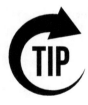

TIP If you are not serving a full meal, you can refer back to the Pairing section for assistance in putting together food trays for your tasting party.

Author's Aside

If you and your guests are up for more of a challenge during the tasting, you can arrange for a blind wine tasting. In this case, guests will not know which wines they are drinking as they taste them. This is done by pouring wines from decanters or covering the bottle/label and letting guests experience the wine before learning the specifics. You can use fabric wine bottle sleeves or other fancy materials. However, I've found that the simple lunch brown bags work perfectly fine. Of course, you will know the wines as they are served so that the tasting order is maintained for the most enjoyable experience.

To up the stakes, you can make it into a contest where guests guess the attributes of the wine. Attributes can include the varietal, the region, the year, or the specific winery. Scores can be kept and prizes (say a bottle of wine) can be given, if you wish.

Enjoying Your Event

When it comes time for your actual wine tasting, you will want to have everything organized and on hand to be able to enjoy the party with your guests. You may need to chill some wines before the official tasting begins, so it is a good idea to start guests with some water (still or mineral) to allow everyone to arrive. Plus, it helps hydrate people and stops them from getting tipsy early on. If you do want to proceed with some glasses of wine as guests arrive, have a bottle or two of sparkling wine or a light white wine chilled and available to start. You will have already decided when a meal will be served, if at all, in relation to the tastings, so simply notify your guests of how the party is scheduled to proceed when they arrive.

If the tasting is covering a variety of wine styles or types (i.e. sparkling and still or whites and reds), you will want to do a short intermission of sorts when transitioning between wine groups. This will allow everyone's palates to clear for a better tasting experience, and will slow down the drinking.

While you can decide to allow guests to pour their own tastings, it is more appropriate to pour wine for each guest. There are two reasons for

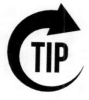

For a wine tasting, the most appropriate amount of wine to pour in a single tasting is 1-2 ounces. An easy way to regulate the pours without getting a measured topper is to simply do a one-one-thousand, two-one-thousand count.

this. One, you are the host, and it is simply more hospitable to offer to pour for those in attendance. Two, you can control the amount of wine served in each glass. This is more critical for larger gatherings, as a standard 750mL wine bottle is only 25 ounces and can only go so far. Every person who wants a tasting should have at least one tasting of each selection of their choosing.

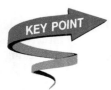

For tasting parties, pour smaller samples of 1-2 ounces to serve more people with a greater selection. A general rule is that one bottle should serve 12 people.

You will organize your tasting wines as follows:

- Light wines are to be served before full-bodied wines (generally whites before reds)

- Drier wines are to be served before sweeter wines

- Lesser-quality wines are to be served before higher-quality wines

- When it comes to red wines, younger vintages are to be served before older vintages.

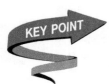

If a guest brings an impressive "WOW" bottle of wine, that is noteworthy or especially pricey, put it at the end of the tasting.

When you are ready to serve a wine for tasting, you will introduce it to your guests (if you are not going blind.) The introduction can include fun facts about the wine from your research and should include the particulars from the label in the form of varietal, winery, location, and year. If you are doing a blind tasting, then you will alert guests as to the type of wine (sparkling, white, red) and leave the trivia element for the end of the tasting when wines' identities are uncovered.

The proper way to participate in a tasting is to wait for everyone to have a sampling of the wine in their glass before sipping. For those who get the early pours, it is easy to use the time it takes for serving everyone as a chance to swirl and to examine the wine as you wait. Some guests may not wait for everyone, but at least you'll know the proper etiquette when you attend a wine tasting. If you are sipping with your guests, serve everyone else first before pouring your glass and setting the bottle aside.

Give your guests time to discuss the wine among themselves or with the group. Remember, it's not a chug-fest. You can help pace everyone. Ask your guests what they see in the wine's color and clarity. Do they see legs in the glass? What do they smell? What tastes do they pick up on? You will probably have people smelling or tasting things in the wine that others do not, so they will continue to taste and discuss.

If a guest requests any additional sample of the wine that was just poured, you can provide more (given that there is any left, of course.) Otherwise, put a partial bottle aside for additional drinking once the official tasting exercise is completed. Let guests know that they can have more of their favorites once the tasting is completed and move on to avoid letting the party get bogged down or letting people overindulge early in the event.

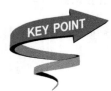

KEY POINT — *As a tasting host, you need to help guests not only enjoy the event but also get home safely.*

The party itself will dictate the overall pace, so allow it to flow as it will. Once the wines for the official tasting are poured, it can become more informal with guests enjoying additional tastings at will. If you find that you have unopened bottles at the event of your party, you can offer them to guests as they leave. Start by offering the person who brought a specific bottle to the party a chance to take it with them, and then open it up to others.

A wine tasting can really be as simple as all of that. The preparation you put into having everything ready beforehand can make the event run smoothly and allow you more of a chance to enjoy the festivities for yourself.

Winery Tastings

The other common wine tasting option comes in the form of visiting a winery to sample wines. You already learned the basics of wine in the previous section, but there are some added points to take into consideration when visiting wineries.

Preparing for a Winery Tour

If you find yourself ready to visit a wine region of any size, you'll want to be prepared. While some wineries have options for purchasing snacks or meals onsite, it is best to bring a picnic of sorts to balance out the wine consumption. What you decide to pack for snacks is a personal preference, but you will definitely want to bring an ample supply of water.

Author's Aside

Here's a little wine country cheat sheet. When traveling to wineries, I typically have an ice chest and a grocery bag filled with food. I will have one or two types of sliced meats (and/or salami) as well as some cheddar and jack cheese. A box of club crackers is a universal way to clear the palate, and sandwich items (bread and spread) can serve for heartier munchies. To keep things simple, I'll get a medium sized container of chopped fruit from the grocery store and maybe some cookies or brownies to sweeten things up. Depending on how many are joining you and how many wineries you will be visiting throughout the day, figure a liter of water per person is the minimum to stay hydrated and maintain a (relatively) clear head.

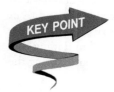 **KEY POINT** *Pack a picnic, snacks, and water when visiting wineries.*

When people first visit wine country the tendency is to try to do too many tastings in a single day or weekend. Wine tasting should be viewed as the proverbial marathon rather than a sprint. If you figure that the typical winery will be tasting 6-8 wines at any one time, that translates into a glass at each stop. Therefore, trying to visit a half dozen wineries in a day is the equivalent to 6 glasses of wine. See why having food with you is handy from both a practical angle and a way to make the experience more enjoyable?

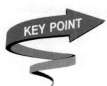 **KEY POINT** *When visiting wine country, develop your transportation strategy before tasting. Do not drink and drive.*

You should expect that a single winery tasting will take about an hour, but it could be longer if you linger. As the day wears on and the number of tastings accumulates, the wines seem "better" at later stops because the alcohol is talking. Personally, I suggest 3 (maybe 4) wineries per day to enjoy the experience and be responsible.

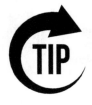

It never hurts to call a given winery before you stop by, to make sure they are open and that there are no special conditions or schedules for tasting. This is especially polite to do if you're traveling a group of six or more. Some wineries require reservations for large parties, but even if it's not required, it's just common courtesy to the service staff, if no one else, to give them a heads-up.

While you can "wing it" when it comes to the wineries you visit, you will most likely have a better experience if you plan your route ahead of time. Wine regions have free maps available in wineries, hotels, and area businesses so that you can get a sense of your options. You can also research wine regions through the internet and get specific directions to and from any of your stops before you embark. It is both a time saver and stress reliever to know where you plan to go ahead of time instead of finding that your desired stops are miles apart and having crisscross the area during the course of your day

///

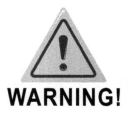

WARNING! Develop your transportation plan before embarking on a tasting. You should establish a designated driver from the start of your day. Most wine regions have a variety of services available for tours or rentals when everyone in your group will be drinking. Do not drink and drive. Law enforcement in wine areas is extra vigilant regarding impaired drivers. Be responsible and make sure the day of wine and fun ends safely.

///

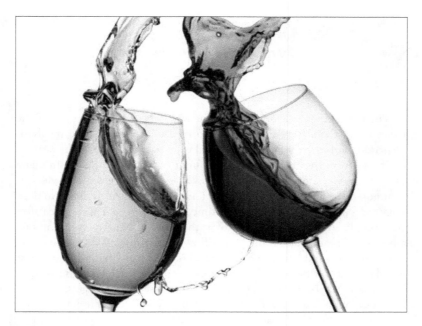

What to Expect at a Winery Tasting

There is no single cookie-cutter winery experience. You could end up in the barrel room of a winery, tasting wine served from a plank sitting between two barrels, while standing with the vineyard dog by your side (these are sometimes the best tastings of them all.) You could also walk into a multi-million dollar tasting room with a full gift shop and restaurant, and there are limitless possibilities between those extremes. The variation is part of the fun.

If you are driving up to a winery and find that the path is dirt or gravel and near any vines, the proper thing to do is to proceed slowly. The reason is that you should avoid kicking up debris into the vines. Usually, signs will be posted to remind you to go slow, but you want to be sure to avoid that mistake.

Author's Aside

It may sound like I'm being a stickler about driving speed, but I have seen people go barreling up to a tasting room, leaving a rooster tail of dust behind them. In two cases, I watched as vineyard owners beelined it to the tasting room and singled out the offenders. The speedy drivers were summarily refused service and bluntly told they weren't welcomed back until they could respect the slower speeds. Yep, it does happen. Remember, you are a guest on the property, and in some cases, that property is actually someone's residence. Drive on their roads as though your own family lived there.

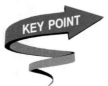

Remember that you are a guest on winery property.
Respect all posted speed limits and other rules.

When you enter a tasting room, you will be greeted with a list of the wines being tasted that day and be notified of any tasting fee involved. Depending on where you are tasting and what you want to sample, tastings can range from free to a general upper limit of five or ten bucks. In many cases, you will be presented with more than one tasting option, which is common if the winery is serving older ("library") wines in addition to their standard wines. The majority of the time, you will pay the tasting fee after you complete the tasting, instead of at the start. In most cases, if you buy a bottle (or more) the tasting fees will also be waived. Wineries institute tasting fees to avoid having people sip and run; after all, they are in business to sell bottles, not individual gulps. Wineries in areas that are popular stops for parties, like bachelorette getaways, will sometimes charge the fee up front because of the number of people who are only there to have a good time on the winery's dime, and have no interest in making a purchase.

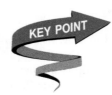

Wine tasting fees are often waived with purchases.

Some wineries offer tasting flights, which are collections of very small sips of many different wines. Typically, a tasting flight will be a series of 1 oz. gulps of different white and red wines. You can choose to taste everything or only the ones that interest you. Also, you can split your tasting with another person, if you want to be able to do more tastings throughout the day without feeling more effect from the alcohol.

The order of the wines served will be arranged for the best tasting experience, so if you want to skip wines, it best to continue down the list. You'll want to rinse your glass between white and red wines. Water and a container to pour everything out will be available on the tasting bar or counter for that purpose. You will also usually find a bowl of crackers or similar items to use between wines to clear your palate.

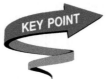

You should taste in the order that wines are listed,
though you can skip those you don't want to try.

Those who work in tasting rooms are very knowledgeable about their products, and they enjoy talking about the wines. Don't be bashful in striking up conversations with staff and other tasters as part of your winery experience. You may be offered additional tastings that were not available on the wine list if you are friendly with the staff. Once you complete the tastings, you may be asked if there are any wines that you would like to revisit. It is a courtesy, not a given. To be polite, do not ask to taste everything again, and do not ask for additional tastes unless you are honestly considering making a purchase of some type.

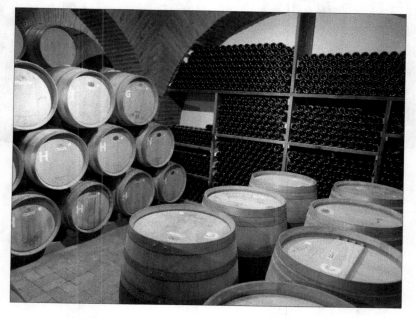

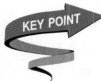 *Tasting at a winery is a social experience. Feel free to talk with the staff and fellow tasters.*

If you are at a larger operation, you may be able to take a tour of the facilities, which can be interesting as you walk through the vines, crush pad, tanks, barrels, and so on. The majority of wineries have areas to sit, picnic and linger, so feel free to take advantage of the opportunity to soak up wine country.

Wineries are in business to sell wines, so you'll more than likely be notified of a wine club of some sort. They take a variety of forms, but typically include a percentage off of purchases as well as a standard shipment of wines throughout the year. Shipments can be frequent (monthly), quarterly, or semi-annual and include a number of bottles in the range of 2-6

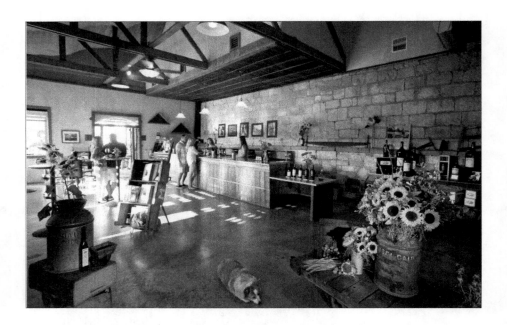

per installment. Wineries will have options for mixed, white only, or red only wine selections. If you like the wines and are willing to make the commitment, they are a great way to stock up on wines that may not be readily available at home. Be sure to understand the terms before signing up regarding the average cost per shipment, timing of shipments, and cancellation policies. Also, be aware that as you visit wineries the tendency to add "just one more" club can come back to haunt you when you receive your credit card bill and the effects of wine are long gone.

TIP Dogs are common traveling companions while visiting wineries. If you are traveling with your dog during your wine tasting excursion, ask the staff in the tasting room about their dog policy prior to taking your dog out of the car. Dogs are welcomed more often than not, but there may be more restrictive policies in effect at specific wineries. Some wineries even have special dog areas and packaged treats for dog visitors. Simply ask first, and be sure that you clean up after your furry friend.

When to Visit a Winery

Just about any time is a good time to visit a winery, in my view. However, depending on what you hope to experience, some times are better than others. Wineries do the most business over the summer weekends, so that is when they are open the longest. Summer is also the busiest time of the year, with the possible exception of harvest events. Once harvest is over in the fall, wineries will tend to open later in the day and close earlier in the evening. If you want more opportunities to taste and don't mind the crowds, then summer is ideal.

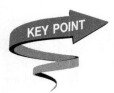

Summer weekends and special events are the busiest times for wineries. They usually have shorter hours in the off season (fall, after harvest, through the winter).

Wine regions will have special festivals or event weekends where there additional activities are available to visitors. For example, at harvest time, many wineries will have winemaker dinners to celebrate the season's yield or events such as bands and fairs to bring guests in to visit. These are fun events, but they are also crowded. You can find out more about events for specific wineries online as nearly all wineries publicize events on their websites and social media.

If the tasting room becomes crowded during your visit, do not monopolize the bar or counter. You can step away to allow others to taste and return to the server for the next pour. The staff sees it all the time. If they don't remember which taste is next, simply remind them. If you don't remember which one is next for you, point to the one you just finished on the menu.

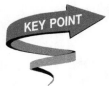

If the tasting room becomes crowded during your visit, do not monopolize the bar or counter. You can step away to allow others to taste and return to the server for the next pour.

If you want a more intimate experience where you get the chance to go at a more leisurely pace and talk more with the staff, you will want to avoid the bigger events. Larger wineries will be open seven days a week, but smaller operations may be closed one or two days a week. If they close, it will usually be on Mondays and/or Tuesdays because those are the least busy. In some cases, they may note that you need to call ahead for tastings. That is usually because they want to be sure someone is in the tasting room, as the staff will otherwise be in the vineyard, so don't think that you're not welcome.

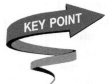

If wineries are not open 7 days a week, the most common days they will be closed are Mondays and Tuesdays.

If you want to experience the vines as well as the wines, you'll want to target early summer through fall for the best visuals. In summer, you will get the lush greens throughout the vineyards. Once there is a cool night or two, the vines will begin to change into the fall colors, with golds and reds.

The choice is yours. Personally, I don't think there's a bad time for a wine country trip. It just depends on what you want to see and do. Different types of opportunities are available to enjoy at wineries during various times of the year.

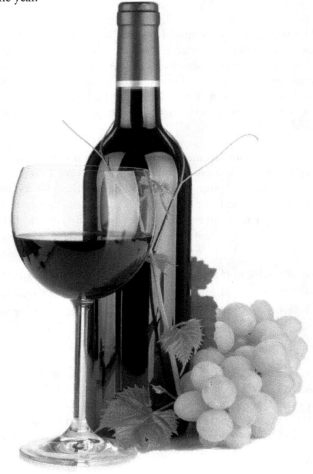

THE TAKEAWAY

Wine tasting can be considered two distinct acts. The first type of wine tasting involves what goes on internally within the wine drinker. To fully appreciate a wine, the tasting experience is a full sensory experience. Wine tasting is also a social activity which is where the second wine tasting distinction is made. Wine tasting in the communal sense can be done in any form and in any place. However, those who love wine often have events centered around vino, which is why it is important to know how to handle the social aspects of wine tasting and winery visits. Once you understand both the internal and social aspects of wine tasting, you can safely assume that you are no longer a true wine beginner; you are officially a wine learner. Welcome to the fun! **Here's your cheat sheet:**

► The mechanics of wine tasting are comprised of the 5 S's: sight, swirl, smell, sip, and swallow/spit.
► When visually examining a wine, look for color and clarity.
► Swirling the wine helps open up the wine to get a better aroma in the glass.
► Swirling a glass should be done by the base or stem of the glass, not the bowl.
► It is completely acceptable to stick your nose into a glass and inhale deeply.
► The aroma will have a variety of characteristics including fruit, herb, spice, floral, and earthy notes.
► The smell of a wine is the aroma and can be referred to as the nose.
► Sipping involves letting the wine roll around in your mouth to get the sensations of taste and texture.
► Different areas of the tongue pick up different elements: sweetness (tip), saltiness (outside edge), acidity (inside edge), and bitterness (back).
► To spit or to swallow wine is a matter of personal choice and preference.
► Once wine has been swallowed or spit out, the wine's aftertaste or finish becomes apparent. A longer finish (30 seconds or more) is desirable for higher quality wines.
► Wine tasting parties can be a fun and relatively easy way to combine learning about wine and socializing.
► Plan to have at least 1 bottle of wine per guest at a tasting party.
► For tasting parties, pour smaller samples of 1-2 ounces to able to serve more people with a greater

selection. A rule of thumb is one bottle should serve 12 people.
► When tasting involves an exceptional ("WOW") wine, serve it last as a Grand Finale to maximize the perception of all wines.
► As a tasting host, you need to help guests not only enjoy the event but also get home safely.
► Pack a picnic, snacks, and water when visiting wineries.
► When visiting wine country, develop your transportation strategy before tasting. Do not drink and drive.
► Remember that you are a guest on winery property. Respect all posted speed limits and other rules.
► Wine tasting fees are often waived with purchases.
► You should taste in the order that wines are listed, though you can skip those you don't want to try.
► Tasting at a winery is a social experience, feel free to talk with the staff and fellow tasters.
► Summer weekends and special events are the busiest times for wineries. They usually have shorter hours in the off season (fall, after harvest, through the winter).
► If the tasting room is crowded, do not monopolize the bar or counter.
► If wineries are not open 7 days a week, the most common days to be closed are Mondays and Tuesdays.

"Wine is one of the most civilized things in the world and one of the most natural things of the world that has been brought to the greatest perfection, and it offers a greater range for enjoyment and appreciation than, possibly, any other purely sensory thing."

—Ernest Hemingway

7

The Wrap

You've come a long way, baby! You can now safely call
yourself a wine lover, rather than a wine beginner. You don't have to
remember it all. You can return to any topic at any time. That's the
beauty of a book...it'll always have your back when you need it.

On the next page, you'll find a compilation of all the key points in
the book. I'd like to leave you with a parting thought—my own oft-stated
quote: "For every wine, there is an occasion, and for every occasion, there is
a wine. Enjoy them all!"

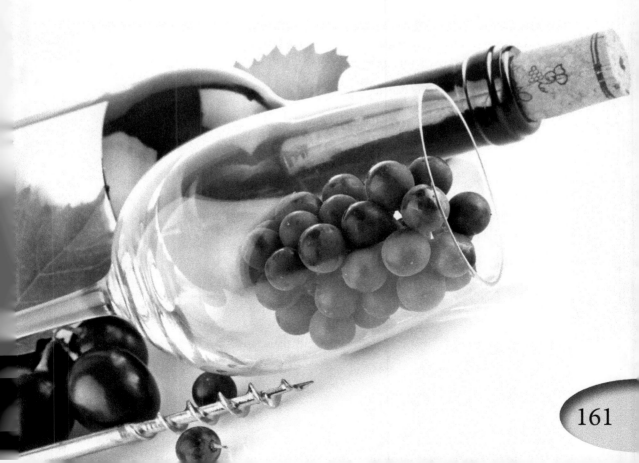

A List of All Key Points In

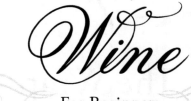

For Beginners

- Wines are generally referred to by either the type of wine, the style that the wine is made, or varietal of grapes used.

- Don't be fooled. White wine can be made from both red and white grapes.

- Rosés are not blends of white and red wine. The color comes from limited contact with grape skins during fermentation.

- The concepts of a blended versus varietal wine can be deceiving. A bottle of Cabernet Sauvignon does <u>not</u> have to be 100% Cabernet Sauvignon.

- The term "Champagne" should only be used to refer to sparkling wines produced in the French region of Champagne.

- Casks range from large vats to barrels, in which wine fermentation and aging occurs. They are typically made of wood or steel.

- Fortified wines contain the addition of distilled spirits, most often brandy.

- Dessert wines are usually sold in smaller bottles due to cost and high levels of sweetness.

- Pinot Gris and Pinot Grigio are from the same grape. Gris is a fuller wine from France, and Grigio is a lighter wine from Italy.

- Chardonnay wines are often characterized by the use of steel or oak during fermentation which can make the wine taste fruitier or more buttery.

- Riesling is a common varietal for late harvest wines. This can lead to the misconception that all Rieslings are super sweet, which is not true.

- Syrah is referred to as Shiraz in Australian wines.

- Syrah and Petite Syrah are not the same grape or wine.

- France and California are considered the biggest players in the world of wine.

- The most notable French wine regions include: Bordeaux, Burgundy, and Champagne.

- The most notable wine regions in California are Napa and Sonoma.

- Other important European regions include the Rhone in France, Germany, Italy, Spain, and Portugal. Oregon, Washington State, and New York are producers in the United States. New World producers include Australia as well as Argentina and Chile in South America.

- Wine can be purchased in grocery stores, specialty shops, wineries, wine bars and lounges, and online.

- Grocery store wine can have a negative connotation due to mass production and the perception of lower quality.

- For white and sparkling wine purchases that will be consumed immediately, chilled bottles may be located in the cooler section of the grocery store.

- When buying online, wine shoppers need to be aware of the local laws governing wine shipments.

- French wines are often labeled with the appellation (geographic origin) rather than the varietal contained in the wine.

- Vintage refers to the year that the grapes used in a wine were harvested. Vintage bottles will lag two or more years due to aging before sale.

- A vintage rating is a broader yardstick than an individual wine rating for determining the likely quality of a bottle of wine.

- Ratings are not universal to all wines of a given year. A good year for one varietal in one region may not be good everywhere.

- Ratings are subjective, based on a critic's tastes.

- Robert Parker is the most recognizable wine critic/wine rating, but other experts do exist.

- Unfiltered wines contain more particles in the wine that are believed to add to the complexity of flavor.

- Organic wines are readily available and are made under strict standards to eliminate or minimize the presence of various chemicals and sulfites.

- Boxed and screw topped wines may be perceived as inferior, but both have benefits that protect wines against damage.

- Wine and cheese pair well for various reasons, most notably because of the balance between sweet and salty components.

- To pair a cheese with a wine, use the acidity and fat content of the cheese as a guide. Light and creamy cheeses tend to go best with white wines. Hard cheeses pair better with red wines.

- As a general rule, white wines go best with seafood, chicken, creamy pasta sauces, and salads.

- As a general rule, red wines pair best with more flavorful pasta sauces, red meats, pork, and chocolates.

- Sparkling wine pairings are not limited to appetizer and dessert trays.

- Pinot Grigio and Pinot Gris are the best matches for salads, vegetables, and seafood.

- Chardonnay pairs well with white meats and flaky and oil seafood.

- Gewürztraminer and Riesling have similar food pairing characteristics and are good for spicy ethnic dishes.

- Pinot Noir can be one of the most versatile red wines for food pairings.

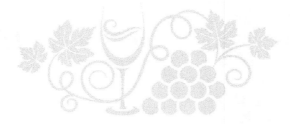

- Merlot wines generally do not pair well with leafy vegetables or seafood but match nicely with tomato-based dishes.

- Zinfandel pairs with meats from turkey to BBQ and cured meats and roasted veggies.

- Cabernet Sauvignon is a compliment to beef and gamier meat dishes as well as all types of chocolate.

- Syrah is the "Big Bad BBQ" wine that overwhelms nearly all vegetables and lighter meat fare.

- Port and dessert wines are not typically served with entrees but can be used as an ingredient in dishes.

- The winged corkscrew is the most common corkscrew used.

- The sommelier knife or wine key is the second most common corkscrew and requires a little more practice to use compared to a winged corkscrew.

- Specialized corkscrews and wine openers are available to assist those who otherwise have difficulty uncorking a bottle.

- Decanting wine is the process of pouring a bottle of wine into a large container before serving in a wine glass.

- Decanters are used to allow sediment in wine to settle before pouring.

- Wine glasses come in a variety of shapes and sizes to maximize the tasting experience of a particular type or style of wine.

- Never "cook" your wine by leaving it in a hot car or other hot environment.

- A partial bottle of sparkling wine should only be recorked with a topper designed specifically for sparkling wines.

- Wine should be stored on its side in a cool, dark environment.

- Wine should be served with a degree of chill based on the type and style.

- Sparkling wines should be served "freezer cold."

- Bottles can be cooled by being placed in the freezer or refrigerator for 30 minutes to 2 hours.

- White wines should be served "refrigerator cold."

- Light red wines should be served "refrigerator cool."

- Bolder red wines should be served "chilled" slightly below room temperature.

- A crumbling cork doesn't mean the wine is automatically ruined, though it can indicate the wine may have a problem from the faulty cork.

- Decanting wine for an hour or so allows the wine to breathe and become more pleasant to drink.

- When deciding which bottle to serve first follow the general guidelines: sparkling wines first; lighter before darker (whites before reds); drier before sweeter; lower quality before higher quality; younger vintages before older vintages (especially for red wines).

- Proper etiquette includes: host first/drink second; ladies first followed by older and honored guests; keep wine within reach for dinner service with multiple bottles if necessary; and offer guests the last sip of wine from a bottle before pouring it for yourself.

- Additional wine options include mimosas, sangria, and mulled wine.

- The mechanics of wine tasting are comprised of the 5 S's: sight, swirl, smell, sip, and swallow/spit.

- When examining the sight of a wine, look for color and clarity.

- Swirling the wine helps open up the wine to get a better aroma in the glass.

- Swirling a glass should be done by the base or stem of the glass, not the bowl.

- It is completely acceptable to stick your nose into a glass and inhale deeply.

- The aroma will have a variety of characteristics from fruit, herb, spice, floral, and earthy notes.

- The smell of a wine is the aroma and can be referred to as the nose.

- Sipping involves letting the wine roll around in your mouth to get the sensations of taste and texture.

- Different areas of the tongue pick up different elements: sweetness (tip), saltiness (outside edge), acidity (inside edge), and bitterness (back).

- To spit or to swallow wine is a matter of personal choice and preference.

- Once wine has been swallowed or spit out, the wine's aftertaste or finish becomes apparent.

- A longer finish (30 seconds or more) is desirable for higher quality wines.

- Wine tasting parties can be a fun and relatively easy way to combine learning about wine and socializing.

- Have one bottle per guest as a general rule. While some will not drink a full bottle during the course of the party, this will ensure that you have enough to cover everyone. Keep a couple extra on hand, as well, in case a guest fails to bring their assigned wine.

- For tasting parties, pour smaller samples of 1-2 ounces to able to serve more people with a greater selection. A rule of thumb is one bottle should serve 12 people.

- If a guest brings an impressive "WOW" bottle of wine, that is noteworthy or especially pricey, put it at the end of the tasting.

- As a tasting host, you need to help guests not only enjoy the event but also get home safely.

- Pack a picnic, snacks, and water when visiting wineries.

- When visiting wine country, develop your transportation strategy before tasting. Do not drink and drive.

- Remember that you are a guest on winery property. Respect all posted speed limits and other rules.

- Wine tasting fees are often waived with purchases.

- You should taste in the order that wines are listed, though you can skip those you don't want to try.

- Tasting at a winery is a social experience, feel free to talk with the staff and fellow tasters.

- Summer weekends and special events are the busiest times for wineries. They usually have shorter hours in the off season (fall, after harvest, through the winter).

- If the tasting room becomes crowded during your visit, do not monopolize the bar or counter. You can step away to allow others to taste and return to the server for the next pour.

- If wineries are not open 7 days a week, the most common days to be closed are Mondays and Tuesdays.

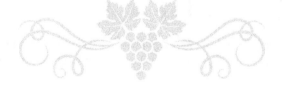

The Deep Dish

In this section, you'll find additional resources and references you may find helpful. That includes other books, web sites, movies and more, as well as a few drink recipes and The Lingo—a glossary of all the Shop Talk (or wine speak) elements you encountered throughout the book.

Below are some of my recommendations to help you continue your exploration of wines and wine resources. ***Enjoy your learning!***

Print: Books

If you are interested in learning more about the history of wine, you may find these reads interesting:

- *Vintage: The Story of Wine*, Hugh Johnson, 1989

- *Uncorked: The Science of Champagne*, Gérard Liger-Belair, 2004

- Elin McCoy, *The Emperor of Wine: The Rise of Robert M. Parker, Jr. and the Reign of the American Taste*, 2005

- *A Short History of Wine*, Rod Phillips, 2000

- *A History of Wine in America, Vol 1: From the Beginnings to Prohibition*, Thomas Pinney, 2007

- *A History of Wine in America, Vol 2: From Prohibition to the Present*, Thomas Pinney, 2007

- *The Oxford Companion to Wine*, Jancis Robinson, 2006

Print: Magazines

- *Wine Spectator*
  This magazine is available in print and online. It is one of the most referenced publications in the wine community. It is oriented towards wine drinkers in the United States.

- *Wine Enthusiast*
  This magazine covers wine news and ratings. The online version is available at www.winemag.com. This publication is more global in focus, as its subtitle "The World in Your Glass" acknowledges.

- *Food & Wine*
  This magazine gives especially useful ideas for food and wine pairings.

Movies

- *Bottle Shock,* 2008
  Hands-down this is my favorite wine movie. It covers the Judgment in Paris where the underdog wines of California's Chateau Mantelena shocked the world by beating French wines in a blind tasting.

- *French Kiss,* 1995
  This is a romantic comedy that does have a wine tie-in. It's an enjoyable "just sit back and enjoy your wine while you watch" movie that is also good date night viewing.

- *A Walk in the Clouds*, 1995
  This romantic, historical piece is set on a Northern California vineyard in the World War II era. It is definitely chick-flick fare, but another film that is made for sipping wine.

- *Sideways*, 2004
  This was a popular movie about men having a bit of a mid-life crisis while exploring the Santa Barbara, California wine scene. Not exactly a personal favorite, but it does have a wine-theme that works for men.

Web

▶ **Overall Outstanding Wine Resource:**

   ♦ **Wine Folly**, Winefolly.com, 2014
   I love this website because of the infographics that make complex concepts easy to understand.

▶ **Information on Wine Terms:**

   ♦ **Glossary**, Wine Spectator, Glossary, 2014

▶ **Information on the History of Wine:**

   ♦ **The Origins and Ancient History of Wine**, University of Pennsylvania Museum of Archeology and Anthropology, 2014

   ♦ **WINE 101: Wine History,** Professional Friends of Wine, Jim LaMar, 2014

   ♦ **The 1976 Paris Tasting,** Stag's Leap, 2014
   This is the history of the "Judgment in Paris" from the perspective of the winery that supplied the winning red wine, as compared to the Bottle Shock movie that follows the winning Chardonnay producer.